POWER OVER PCOS:

THE 7 STEP SOLUTION FOR POLYCYSTIC OVARY SYNDROME

JULIE MERRICK
ND BHSC

Title: Power Over PCOS: The 7 Step Solution For Polycystic Ovary Syndrome
ISBN: 978-1-921681-35-6 (pbk.)

Published by Book Pal
www.bookpal.com.au

www.poweroverpcosbook.com

DISCLAIMER:

Acknowledgements

This book has been a long time coming, and I would firstly like to thank my website subscribers for their patience in awaiting both the e-book, and now the printed version of my book Power Over PCOS. I also appreciate the many thank you emails I have received, and I'm grateful to those who have participated in my research surveys.

Many thanks go to the mentors and coaches I've had over the years, and those who have taught me how to get my message across, especially through the medium of the internet. These include Wayne Pickstone, Steve Baker, Lorraine Mill, Adam Gibson, Pete Godfrey, Darren Stephens, and Andrew and Daryl Grant.

I would also like to thank my colleagues at the Blue Mountains Wellness Centre, and the group of fantastic natural health professionals I have had the pleasure of getting to know over the past couple of years who have encouraged, advised, and congratulated me on my journey.

Lastly, thank you to my parents and family, who have encouraged me to pursue this journey, and provided unconditional support (and lots of babysitting!). And thank you Jay for being my number one inspiration.

About The Author

Julie Merrick is a naturopath who holds a Health Science degree in Complementary Medicine, is a member of the Australian Natural Therapists Association, and is a professional member of the Polycystic Ovarian Syndrome Association of Australia.

After running two successful clinics in the Blue Mountains of Australia helping patients with a wide variety of conditions, she now dedicates her time to helping women around the world with polycystic ovary syndrome. After her own experience with PCOS and her success in overcoming the challenges it brings, she created the 7 Step Solution so she could help other women achieve results like hers.

Knowing there was a limit to how many women she could help face to face, she collated her knowledge and created an online program that takes women through her 7 Step Solution week by week. In 2008 she was publicly acknowledged among her peers for her achievements with this by winning the Best of the Best award at the Global Wellness Summit in Queensland.

Julie believes that to achieve true healing, you must identify and target the underlying factors that lead to your symptoms, rather than just treating the symptoms themselves. She also believes in taking a holistic approach by addressing the physical, structural, environmental, and emotional contributors to ill health, and supporting the body's natural healing process.

Julie provides regular PCOS tips and newsletters for over 7000 subscribers at www.poweroverpcos.com, and is available for personal guidance through her online PCOS Success System at www.pcossuccess.com.

Contents

SECTION ONE

ALL ABOUT PCOS

What is it and why do I have it?

PCOS – WHAT IS IT?

Polycystic ovary syndrome, or PCOS, is a hormonal and metabolic disorder affecting women. It is so named because of the multiple cyst like structures in the ovaries of many women with the condition.

These cysts are actually follicles; fluid filled structures that don't fully mature in the ovaries because of a lack of ovulation. Despite the name, not all women with PCOS have polycystic ovaries, although most do. The cysts are just one of the many manifestations that can occur in PCOS.

→ *In a POWER over PCOS survey of over 200 women, 73% of respondents said they had multiple cysts on the ovaries, as discovered by ultrasound, 14% did not have polycystic ovaries but had symptoms of PCOS, and 13% had not had an ultrasound.*

PCOS disrupts normal hormonal balance, and normal blood sugar regulation. It can result in weight gain and fertility problems, menstrual problems, and also skin and hair problems.

It is associated with impaired glucose tolerance, or insulin resistance, and often involves high androgen levels in the blood. Several other abnormalities can occur, which will be discussed shortly.

Polycystic ovaries can also be found in women who don't have polycystic ovary syndrome, making the name of this condition rather misleading. Some women just have PCO, the cysts without any of the symptoms that make up the syndrome.

PCOS affects a woman's appearance, metabolism, and femininity, and can result not only in physical symptoms, but many psychological issues such as anxiety, depression, relationship problems, and eating disorders. Many women say they feel like 'half a woman', or that they 'hate looking in the mirror', and consequently, many women with PCOS have quite low self esteem. Many also feel that their body is letting them down.

Effectively managing PCOS is important for both the physical health of the woman, and her psychological wellbeing.

WHAT ARE THE SYMPTOMS?

PCOS can manifest a variety of symptoms, and it is important to mention that the syndrome varies greatly between different women. You do not need to have all of the following symptoms to have PCOS. For example, many women with PCOS are overweight, but some are of normal weight or even slightly underweight.

PCOS symptoms:

- Weight gain, especially around the abdomen
- Difficulty losing weight
- Scalp hair loss
- Hirsutism - Excess male pattern hair growth. E.g.: facial hair, excess body hair
- Acne on the face or body, especially around the jaw line
- Irregular menstrual cycles (oligomenorrhea)
- Absent periods
- Lack of ovulation, trouble conceiving
- Skin tags – small growths of skin, often found in the armpits or skin folds
- Acanthosis nigricans – darkened patches of skin around skin folds
- Multiple cystic follicles in the ovary

- Sweet cravings or excess hunger
- Sleepiness after meals
- Mood swings, anxiety, depression
- Recurrent miscarriages

In addition to the main symptoms of PCOS, some women also experience:

- Heavy or painful periods
- Endometriosis
- A deeper voice
- Dizziness
- Eating disorders
- Underactive thyroid gland
- Asthma
- Recurrent thrush
- Fatigue
- Digestive problems
- Gestational diabetes

WHAT CAUSES PCOS AND ITS SYMPTOMS?

Most of the symptoms of PCOS are caused by elevated insulin levels and testosterone levels, combined with a variety of other hormonal abnormalities that vary among women. Some have high prolactin levels, high luteinizing hormone (LH), low follicle stimulating hormone (FSH), low progesterone, and oestrogen dominance (high oestrogen in relation to progesterone).

High testosterone levels cause masculinisation, and contribute to symptoms such as acne and excess hair. However, some women have normal levels of testosterone and still experience skin and hair problems. In these cases, it is possible that there is an increased *sensitivity* of the tissues to testosterone which is causing the symptoms, rather than elevated levels. There may also be other factors contributing to these symptoms, such as nutrient deficiencies. High testosterone also disrupts the delicate balance of other hormones required for a normal menstrual cycle, and can contribute to irregular cycles and a lack of ovulation.

Higher than normal levels of the hormone insulin are common and insulin resistance is one of the proposed causes of PCOS symptoms. Insulin is the hormone that stimulates the transport of sugar or glucose, into the cells from the bloodstream. Over time, when high levels of insulin are consistently produced, the insulin receptors on cell walls become down-regulated, meaning they reduce in number or become less responsive to insulin's effects.

Because they have become 'resistant' to insulin, more insulin is often produced to try and encourage the blood sugar to enter the cells, but further resistance can then occur, creating a vicious cycle!

The persistent high levels of insulin interfere with the burning of fat for energy, making it difficult to lose weight. It also stimulates the production of testosterone and oestrogen from the ovaries, which in turn stimulates the pituitary gland to release LH, the hormone that normally triggers ovulation. You would think this would be a good thing, considering PCOS often involves a reduced ability to ovulate, but the LH levels usually stay elevated because of this constant stimulation, and this encourages even more testosterone production! Overall, the effects of high insulin are complex but crucial in the pathophysiology of polycystic ovary syndrome.

Insulin resistance can also be the reason why skin tags and dark skin patches occur, usually in areas where the skin folds, like the armpits, groin, and neck. Skin tags, or acrochordon, are small elevated lumps of skin, they may be normal skin colour, or slightly darker than the rest of the skin, and are not known to be cancerous. It is unsure exactly why they appear, but may result from the effects of either high insulin which acts as a growth promoter, or high blood sugar which interferes with normal cell structures.

Polycystic ovaries (multiple follicles) develop when ovulation repeatedly does not occur. A follicle in the ovary normally releases an egg for fertilisation approximately once per month. This occurs in the middle of a menstrual cycle, but in women with PCOS, this does not always happen. The follicle stays put and does not release an egg, and another follicle starts to grow in preparation for ovulation. This creates an effect like a string of pearls which can be seen on ultrasound, and sometimes can lead to enlargement of the ovaries.

Normally after an egg is released, the remaining structure, now called the *corpus luteum*, produces the hormone progesterone which matures the lining of the uterus in preparation for a possible pregnancy. When ovulation does not occur, no corpus luteum is formed, which leads to lower levels of progesterone in women with PCOS.

Many women with PCOS complain of excessive hunger or sweet cravings, often in the afternoon and evenings. This can occur because of insulin resistance, which means that less blood sugar makes its way into the cells for energy. This creates more hunger, especially for sugar or carbohydrate rich foods, in an attempt to bring more sugar into the cells. Sweet cravings can also occur with a poor diet, high in foods that cause a rapid rise and fall in blood glucose.

Fatigue and sleepiness after meals is a common consequence of high insulin levels or insulin resistance. Because the cells become starved of sugar in a sense, it is the cells that become fatigued, because they have less sugar to help produce energy. Sleepiness after meals can also be caused by the uptake of tryptophan by the brain, in response to high insulin. Tryptophan is an amino acid that is a precursor for serotonin, a chemical that is involved in the production of melatonin, the sleep hormone. Because insulin is a hormone that encourages growth, it causes the mobilisation of amino acids like tryptophan to be used for protein synthesis which is the building of new cells, molecules, and cell structures.

Mood swings are common in PCOS and insulin resistance, and are likely to be from both cause and effect. Metabolic and hormonal imbalances can affect brain function, mood, and behaviour, and the distress caused by the symptoms of PCOS can in themselves cause mood swings and psychological effects.

Miscarriage can occur more often in women with PCOS who become pregnant. This may be due to a combination of factors such as low progesterone, which makes the uterine lining less 'mature' and less able to support the implantation of an embryo. It has also been linked with high testosterone levels, and insulin resistance. Women with PCOS who have elevated LH levels are also more likely to suffer a miscarriage[1]. Another possibility is that it may due to blood flow problems and inflammation in which the blood is more viscous, affecting normal blood flow to the uterus and placenta. Miscarriage can also occur because of factors not associated with PCOS such as a genetic abnormality in the foetus, or lifestyle factors involving the mother such as a smoking habit. High caffeine intake of more than 200mg a day has also been found to contribute to an increased risk of miscarriage[2].

It is more likely that a combination of factors is responsible for the development of PCOS rather than a single cause. Insulin resistance, genetic susceptibility, environmental toxins, poor diet and lifestyle, and also chronic low grade inflammation have all been implicated.

My views on the causes of PCOS and the causes of all states of imbalance in the body will be discussed in section two, followed by natural solutions for dealing with these causes, to allow you to gain control over PCOS and your overall health and wellbeing.

HOW IS IT DIAGNOSED?

To confirm a diagnosis of suspected PCOS, tests can be performed to check for common abnormalities that may occur in PCOS, and also to rule out other causes for your symptoms. For example, some other conditions such as congenital adrenal hyperplasia, Cushing's syndrome, hypothyroidism, tumours of the pituitary, adrenal glands, and ovaries, can produce symptoms that can mimic PCOS. Some medications can also produce symptoms associated with PCOS, so it is important to have a thorough medical evaluation to determine what is causing your symptoms and whether it is actually PCOS.

PCOS is usually diagnosed based on the combined presence of symptoms and abnormalities in blood tests. The most common symptoms are menstrual irregularities or a lack of periods, excess hair growth, and weight gain. But as mentioned previously, the symptoms can vary greatly between women. The most common blood tests performed are:

- Testosterone or free androgen index (FAI) – usually high end of normal or high
- Sex hormone binding globulin (SHBG) – usually low end of normal or low
- Glucose tolerance test (GTT) – usually shows impaired glucose tolerance or insulin resistance

- Luteinizing hormone (LH) – can be high in some women
- Follicle stimulating hormone (FSH) – normal to low

In addition, you may be tested for:

- Oestradiol
- Progesterone
- 17-hydroxyprogesterone
- Prolactin
- Cholesterol
- Triglycerides (can be high in PCOS)
- Thyroid stimulating hormone (TSH)
- Glucose (to detect diabetes)
- DHEAS (can be normal to high in PCOS)
- Homocysteine (can be high in PCOS)

Your doctor will evaluate these results in combination with your symptom history to determine if you have PCOS. An ultrasound is useful but not essential to support a diagnosis.

Tests are useful not only to diagnose PCOS but to evaluate your state of health and enable monitoring of treatments to ensure they are working. They can also indicate if you are at risk of certain complications such as heart disease or diabetes. I will be discussing a larger variety of tests you can get from your doctor and naturopath in more detail in section three.

ARE THERE ANY RISKS IN HAVING PCOS?

PCOS can make you more prone to developing certain conditions, but the degree of risk is dependent on the severity of your symptoms such as anovulation and infrequent periods, obesity, and insulin resistance. The main risk seems to be for the development of Type 2 diabetes, the precursor for which is insulin resistance. Type 2 diabetes occurs when the pancreas starts to fail in its production of the hormone insulin. Consequently, blood sugar levels rise because there is not enough insulin to help sugar exit the bloodstream and enter the cells. Symptoms such as thirst and increased urination can occur.

Type 2 diabetes is greatly preventable, following a healthy diet and doing regular exercise is the basis for this prevention but there is a lot more that can be done, which will be discussed in section three.

A woman with PCOS who becomes pregnant may also be at an increased risk for gestational diabetes, which is a temporary diabetes that occurs during pregnancy. Miscarriage can also be more likely in women with PCOS.

If a woman with PCOS has a lack of, or infrequent periods with infrequent ovulation, her progesterone levels will be lower than optimal. This, combined with unopposed oestrogen can make the uterine lining thicker than it should be (endometrial hyperplasia), which over time may increase the risk for endometrial cancer developing. Regular periods cause shedding of this uterine lining, preventing it from thickening, and progesterone helps to 'mature' the lining and also prevent the thickening caused by oestrogen.

Proper management of PCOS will ensure adequate progesterone levels and regular periods of shedding to help prevent this possible complication.

Other complications may occur, not necessarily as a direct result of having PCOS, but from a combination of factors that may be associated with PCOS.

With severe insulin resistance and the development of diabetes, cardiovascular risk factors can also manifest, such as high blood pressure, high blood cholesterol, large waist circumference, and high triglycerides. These factors increase the risk for heart disease and strokes.

Women with PCOS who are overweight may also be prone to the development of sleep apnoea, a serious condition in which breathing is interrupted many times each night, often without any awareness of what is happening. Sleep apnoea also increases your risk of heart problems and strokes, and worsens insulin resistance. Daytime sleepiness is the most common symptom, and many sufferers report waking with a dry mouth, or have high blood pressure that is not managed well on medication.

Alzheimer's disease is another possible complication of PCOS, again, not directly, but through other risk factors such as being overweight and having insulin resistance. Inflammation has also been implicated in the development of Alzheimer's, as it has with PCOS and heart disease.

These increased risks may sound scary and overwhelming, but the majority of risks that may be associated with PCOS are very much preventable. Through having this knowledge you can take steps to maximize your health and help prevent these conditions from developing.

INTERESTING STATISTICS

According to a POWER over PCOS survey,

- **85% of women with PCOS want to lose weight**

- **75% are tired most of the time**

- 59% feel ugly and hate looking in the mirror

- 75% have had a negative experience with a medical professional (eg: being told that PCOS is not a real medical condition....only a cosmetic problem, being told they will never have children or never be able to lose weight, or there's nothing they can do, just come back when you want to try conceiving)

- 75% also suffer with additional symptoms such as headaches, migraines, dizziness, excess sweating, bowel problems, and insomnia.

- 48% have emotional eating problems or eating disorders

- 81% experience regular sugar or carbohydrate cravings

- 46% don't eat breakfast

- 20% have been diagnosed with sleep apnoea

These are concerning statistics. The physical and emotional effects of PCOS should not be underestimated. It is a major health issue for many women, and education for both patients and health professionals are the key to achieving better outcomes.

PROS AND CONS OF SOME MEDICAL TREATMENTS

Figure 1:

Medication:	Benefits:	Possible Disadvantages:
Metformin (also diaformin, glucophage)	Improvement in insulin sensitivity. Lower blood glucose and insulin levels.	• Reduced levels of Vitamin B12 and Folic acid. • Gastrointestinal upset • Risk of lactic acidosis
Clomid (clomiphene citrate)	Stimulates ovulation to increase chance of conception.	• Hot Flushes • Abdominal discomfort • Ovarian enlargement • Birth defects
Oral Contraceptive Pill (OCP)	Reduction in acne, excess hair. Regular cycles. Contraceptive.	• Possible blood clots • Fluid retention • Some OCPs increase insulin resistance, a risk factor for type 2 diabetes • Mood changes • Gastrointestinal upset • Headaches • Reduced levels of Vitamins C, B2, B5, B6, B12, folic acid, and zinc, magnesium, and tryptophan. Especially with long term use. • Reduction in beneficial bacteria in the digestive tract.
Roaccutane for acne (isotretinoin)	High success rate in clearing acne	• Birth defects • Dry, flaky, sensitive skin • Dryness & irritation in

		gastrointestinal tract • Risk of liver abnormalities • Possible risk of mood swings and depression (unproven) • Cannot undergo waxing treatments as some skin will come off
Antibiotics for acne	Reduction in acne	• Gastrointestinal upset • Thrush • Reduction of beneficial gut bacteria • Reduction in vitamin K & biotin production • Lowered immune function
Spironolactone (e.g.: aldactone, an anti-androgen and diuretic)	Reduction in excess hair growth and acne	• Menstrual irregularities • Gastrointestinal upset • Lethargy • Headache • Confusion

If you are taking any of the above medications, seek advice about taking supplements to reduce the nutrient depletion that may occur. If you are experiencing side effects, see section three for some natural solutions to dealing with the common side effects associated with these medications.

CAN IT BE MANAGED NATURALLY?

Absolutely, I am living proof, and that is why I wrote this book, to educate you about how to optimise your health and manage your PCOS symptoms. Your body is intelligent; it knows what to do to regulate its own functioning when given the right tools to do it.

SECTION TWO

WHY ME?

*How did I get this and
what can I do about it?*

Getting diagnosed with PCOS can be both frightening and a relief. Frightening in the sense that you have a 'medical condition' that may cause diabetes, heart disease, or make it difficult to have children, and yet a relief in that you now have a name for all the troubling symptoms you have been experiencing, and that you are not the only one out there with this condition.

When the symptoms get overwhelming, as I know they can, you often find yourself thinking "Why me?", or "How did I get this?" And more importantly, "What can I do about it?" This section of the book will explain the whys and the hows behind PCOS, your symptoms, and ill health in general. It will also explain my controversial view that Insulin Resistance is NOT in fact the root cause of PCOS. Although it *is* one of the causes of your *symptoms*, you will see that the origin of PCOS does not begin with insulin resistance, and is therefore not the root cause.

I encourage you to read and understand this section very well before reading the POWER over PCOS Protocol in section three. The reason is, before knowing the best ways to help PCOS, you need to understand about the different models of health care we have, and how the western health care system which is more appropriately named as the 'disease-care system', does not have the complete answers to help you deal with PCOS. You will understand that a change in mindset and a paradigm shift from 'disease treatment' to 'wellness promotion' is needed, and that an integrated approach to health care is the best way to achieve positive outcomes for patients.

Mostly, you will finally understand how you got to be in the state that you are in today, and you will realise that the best healer available to help you is in fact your own body.

The following information will take you on a journey of discovery into how your state of health becomes disrupted, how disease develops, and how overcoming your condition and achieving amazing health is well within your reach......

HEALTH CARE SYSTEMS

Medical Model of health care

The western medical system is based on the treatment of disease and symptoms by way of pharmaceutical drugs, surgery, and other treatments such as radiation therapy. The emergence of new medical technology and pharmaceuticals has been responsible for many positive advancements in health care, especially with infectious diseases and emergency life saving procedures. It excels in diagnostics and acute care.

The medical model has some disadvantages however, mainly involving the risks and side effects of drugs, and the actual medical system itself. Hospitals are understaffed and over-worked, general practitioners don't have enough time with their patients, the focus is on the disease itself and not the 'whole' person, and in certain countries the financial expense of a trip to hospital is huge, especially for the uninsured. The medical model has become a tug of war between politics, financial gain, and health.

Drugs form the main part of the medical model. Because this form of medicine is now considered mainstream, we have become accustomed to thinking that if we have a symptom, we need to take a drug for it. Pharmaceutical drugs by definition are actually a controlled poison. For a substance to be approved as a drug, it has to achieve an Ld50. This means that the authorities have to know the amount of the drug that will cause death in 50% of the subjects it is tested on (animals, usually rats). Once this lethal dose is discovered, studies can be done to determine a 'therapeutic' dose that is considered safe and effective for humans.

However, several drugs that were once considered safe have now been taken off the market due to serious side effects or an increased risk of death. The medical model is not foolproof, there is no way you can really determine how safe a drug will be unless you try it on humans for a long period of time. Who wants to be a lab rat?

Having said this, there are many medications that have greatly improved quality of life for many people. They are beneficial when used correctly and when the benefits outweigh the risks and side effects. The problem is that many people have to take an additional drug to combat the side effects of the other drug, and then another drug to combat the side effects of the drug that was prescribed to stop the side effects of the first drug! Unfortunately, many people each year fall victim to the negative effects of drugs. In fact, over 100,000 people a year die from properly prescribed medications! [4] Ironically, that makes the medical system, a system designed to combat disease, a major cause of death itself!

TOP CAUSES OF DEATH:

In 2002, the National Vital Statistics Report stated the number of deaths from each of the following causes:

1. Heart disorders: 710,760 deaths
2. Malignant neoplasms (cancer): 553,091
3. Iatrogenic (medical system): 225,000 (averaged from previous data)
4. Cerebrovascular diseases (e.g.: stroke): 167,661
5. Chronic lower respiratory diseases: 122,009

The 225,000 deaths attributed to the medical system are further broken down into the following causes:

- 12,000 -- unnecessary surgery
- 7,000 -- medication errors in hospitals
- 20,000 -- other errors in hospitals
- 80,000 -- infections in hospitals
- 106,000 -- non-error, negative effects of drugs

Although these statistics are shocking and very concerning, I am not anti-medicine. In fact, I was going to go down this route as a career choice, but I changed my mind when I realised, through researching and my own personal experiences, how much of an impact I could have on health by educating people about the 'Wellness' model of health care.

What I *am* against though, is the over-reliance on pharmaceuticals in health care, and the lack of emphasis on prevention and nutrition. There are prevention strategies in place within the medical system, but many of them involve 'false prevention' such as vaccinations and early detection tests. Early detection is great if you unknowingly have a disease, but it is not true prevention.

The medical system excels in acute care and emergency treatments. If I had a broken bone or a life threatening illness, I would not want to go to the local health food store! When there is an acute or serious situation, your best bet is your local doctor or hospital, but with chronic conditions, I believe nature knows best. People need to be educated on how to maximise their health, and not be brought up to believe that if you have a symptom, you need to take a drug for it.

NATUROPATHIC OR WELLNESS MODEL OF HEALTH CARE

The naturopathic or wellness model of health care is focused both on the treatment and prevention of ill health, using nutrition and natural substances in conjunction with, or as opposed to drugs. It is based on the fact that the body knows how to heal itself, when given the right environment.

It aims to encourage innate healing processes, and works with the body, not against it. It aims to provide a strong foundation of health rather than just treating symptoms. We believe that the body is intelligent and it wants to be healthy. Most people, when they suffer with a disease, think that their body has turned against them, but in fact it is doing the opposite. It is looking out for you, trying to tell you that something needs attention.

The wellness model aims to provide the body with optimum levels of all nutrients, a healthy balanced diet and lifestyle, a good attitude, and a respect for nature. I truly believe that we would not be put on this earth without means for survival and good health. I also believe that plants were not just put on this earth to look pretty. The power of nature's pharmacy should not be underestimated, and should not be sidelined as 'grandma's home remedies', but a valid and effective form of medicine that is available to everyone. Before the advent of drug manufacture, natural medicine was the *only* form of medicine, the 'traditional medicine' of society. *Drug* based treatments are really the 'new age' medicine, and not the other way round!

This form of medicine is often considered 'alternative' medicine. But I don't believe this is the right word to use. For example, a major part of naturopathic medicine is nutrition.

Nutrition is not alternative! It is a basic and fundamental factor in sustaining life! An alternative treatment should really be classed as something that is used *instead* of the body's own resources. The body is the best healer you have available to yourself, use it!

INTEGRATED MODEL OF HEALTH CARE

An integrated approach allows you to get the best from both worlds. It focuses on using a combination of treatments or therapies to look after the needs of the individual, and takes into account ALL aspects of health, not just the symptoms. For example, rather than just taking a drug for an ailment, you might still decide to take the drug to gain control over the symptoms, but not without addressing all the other things that affect your health, and investigating all other available options. The basic options included in the integrated model include:

1. Diet & Nutrition

2. Lifestyle – healthy habits, sleep, social factors..etc

3. Exercise

4. Natural supplements and plant medicines

5. Mind-Body Medicine & Energy Therapies

6. Structural Integrity & Physical Therapies

7. Drugs

8. Surgery

The first 6 are *necessary* for optimal health. We need a healthy diet & lifestyle, we need to be active, we need to supplement our diet these days, we need our physical structure to be optimal, and we need to have a healthy mind and attitude to fully experience optimal health. Drugs and surgery treat diseases and symptoms, but they are not a basic *need* or *requirement* by the body to sustain health (excluding emergency medicine and surgery for life threatening conditions of course). People can become deficient in nutrients, and can be lacking in physical activity, but you cannot be lacking or deficient in a pharmaceutical drug. They should not be the first choice for a chronic condition such as PCOS, but an option that is available if necessary.

Awareness of the integrated model allows you to be proactive in your health care, and realize that you have CHOICES. It is not a case of saying "I have PCOS, what is *the treatment* for that?", it is a case of saying "I have PCOS, what can I *do* to improve my health and reduce my symptoms?".
Using the integrated model, you can make sure you are doing everything possible to alleviate your condition. For example, say you have a symptom that is troubling you such as headaches. Instead of just taking pain killers regularly to relieve your headaches, you can look at whether any dietary factors are affecting your headaches.

For example, maybe you are not drinking enough water and your headaches are caused by dehydration, or maybe you need to take a magnesium supplement, as magnesium deficiency can often present as headaches. Perhaps your lifestyle is to blame, not enough exercise, or you might be experiencing transient caffeine withdrawal. Your spine could be out of proper alignment which can cause headaches in some cases, so an osteopath or chiropractor can assess this and treat if needed. Maybe your headaches are a symptom of stress and you need to work on this as well.

Can you see how it is important to look for under-recognised causes and solutions to a problem, rather than continuing to mask the symptom with a pain reliever? Your headache is not from a paracetamol deficiency, but it may be from another underlying deficiency or problem. Of course, headaches can also be caused by more serious conditions as well, so it is all the more important to look for causes rather than masking the symptoms.

CAUSES OF DISEASE (INCLUDING PCOS)

Very rarely can a disease be traced back to one specific cause. Usually a combination of factors is involved, and therefore, a disease should not be *treated* by one specific remedy.

In the following pages, you are going to discover how a disease such as PCOS can develop, and how various factors combine to trigger changes in your body that produce symptoms. So, if you have been wondering "Why me?" read on.

Some might say that insulin resistance is the root cause of PCOS, and indeed it contributes to many of the symptoms, **but** *what actually causes the insulin resistance in the first place?* **Ever wondered about that?** You might think that it is your family history and genetics that has caused your PCOS, but did you know that your genes do not actually get the final say as to what happens in your body? That's right; your genes do not have complete control over your health. More on that later...

First of all, it is important to point out that the human body is an intelligent design; it knows what needs doing and how to do it, every second of every day. We sometimes forget how amazing we human beings are! Just the fact that our hearts can continue to beat day in and day out without rest is remarkable.

Every function that occurs in the body that you may take for granted, like breathing, digestion, facial expressions, and moving around, is all the result of a complex orchestration of events involving multiple systems in the body, and most people go through life unaware of the amazing power they have within themselves.

You might be thinking, well that's all well and good, but how can I feel grateful for my body when it is giving me all these horrible symptoms! That's understandable, and I've been there, but let me tell you that 'every sign or symptom in your body is a warning sign of some internal imbalance'. Your body is trying to tell you something and it is time to learn how to listen to what it is saying. Most of all, you need to understand that **PCOS is not something you have to 'fight', you have to look at why your symptoms are occurring and take action to work 'with' your body not against it. You need to take proactive steps to improve your body's internal environment, so that your body is in an optimal state of health to be able to function the way it was designed.**

WHERE DOES IT ALL START?

The origin of diseases such as PCOS can be summarized into 6 steps, each step building on the previous one. Before I go into detail, the following diagram summarises the basics of these 6 consecutive steps:

Figure 2

ORIGINS OF DISEASE

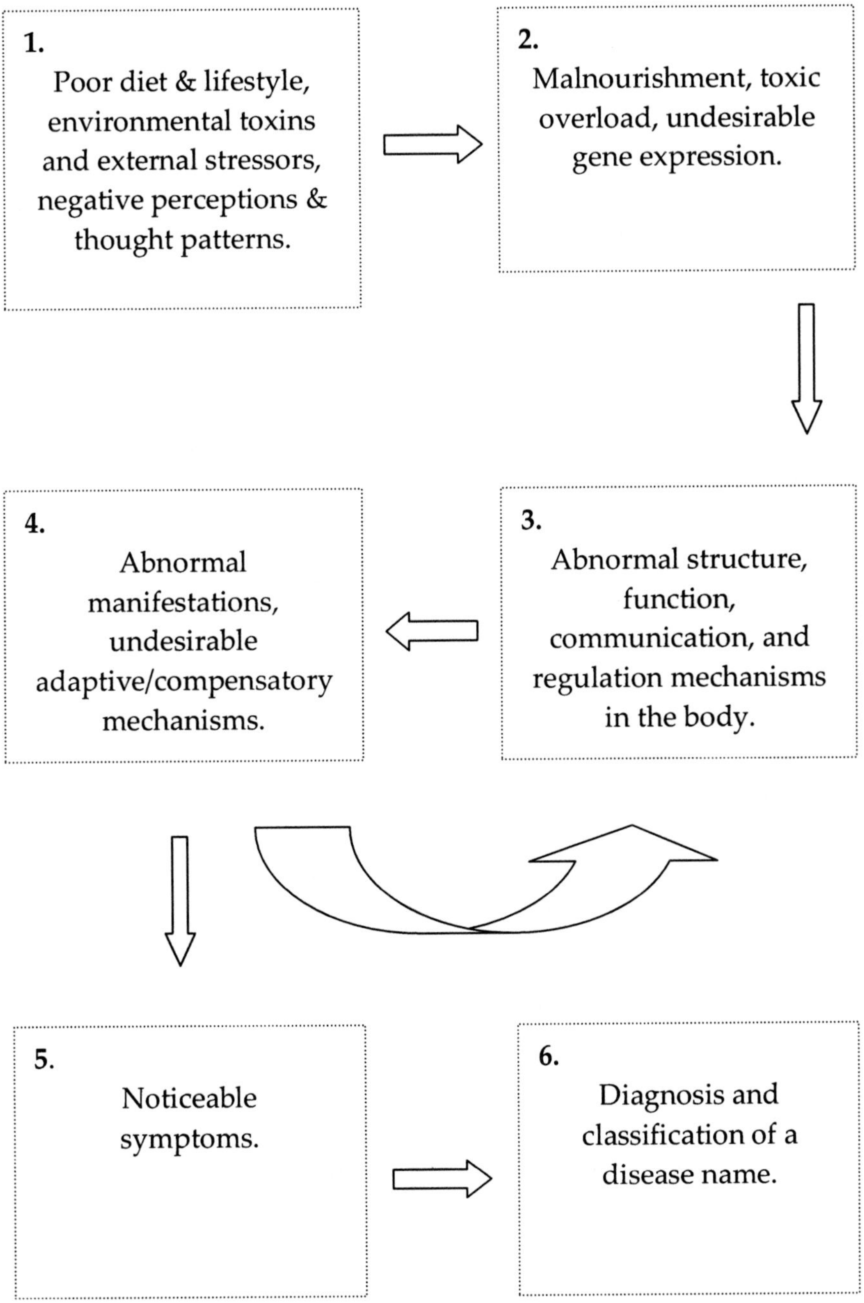

1.
Poor diet & lifestyle, environmental toxins and external stressors, negative perceptions & thought patterns.

2.
Malnourishment, toxic overload, undesirable gene expression.

4.
Abnormal manifestations, undesirable adaptive/compensatory mechanisms.

3.
Abnormal structure, function, communication, and regulation mechanisms in the body.

5.
Noticeable symptoms.

6.
Diagnosis and classification of a disease name.

HOW EACH STEP LEADS TO THE NEXT:

1. Poor diet and lifestyle, environmental toxins and external stressors, perceived stress and negative thought patterns.

Examples:

- Poor food choices
- Poor food quality
- Overeating
- Alcohol
- Reduced nutrient content in soil
- Green harvesting
- Food storage and processing
- Synthetic food additives
- Pesticides...etc
- Plastics
- Pollution
- Smoking
- Radiation
- Household chemicals
- Synthetic personal care and cosmetic products
- Medications & drugs
- Lack of sufficient or appropriate exercise
- 24 hour lifestyle, less relaxation, more pressures
- Poor sleep habits
- Negative perceptions and attitudes, limiting beliefs

1.

a) Poor diet and lifestyle:

It is well known that a healthy diet and lifestyle has a positive influence on a person's health. Our state of health is a direct result of how we live, combined with our genetics and our perceptions and attitude. When looking to improve your health, one of the first and most basic places to start is with your diet. When I say diet, I don't mean a 'diet' as such, like a weight loss program or a restrictive eating plan. I use the term diet to mean the types, quantity, and quality of foods that you eat each day.

Your food and fluid intake does more than just provide energy and keep you alive, it provides the building blocks for your cells and the nutrients for your cells to function and perform the millions of vital processes in the body. Your body needs many different types of nutrients each day to function, if any are deficient or missing, your cells will not function properly and your state of health will be affected. Therefore, poor dietary choices and subsequent multiple nutrient deficiencies can directly contribute to impaired functioning in the body, which paves the way for disease processes to be initiated.

In the twenty first century, our food quality is not what it used to be fifty or so years ago. Due to modern farming practices such as pesticide use, green harvesting (when plant foods are picked while unripe), long periods of transport and storage (sometimes up to a year), and rapid artificial ripening of foods to make them ready for sale, the nutrient content of our food has declined. Some nutrients only develop in the food in the last twenty four to forty eight hours of natural ripening. Picking food when green and artificially ripening them does not allow time for the full range of nutrients to develop. It might look normal in the grocery store, but looks can be deceiving.

A good example is with tomatoes. Have you noticed that tomatoes these days are very firm and often pale on the inside? Those who are old enough to remember will say that tomatoes from years ago were softer and richer in colour and taste. That is because the nutrients are responsible for these characteristics.

Even foods that are vine-ripened may not have their full nutrient content due to the soil becoming more and more depleted of nutrients. This is because of the lack of crop rotation, and land is not left to lie fallow between harvests. New crops are planted right away to meet demands of mass production, leaving little time for the soil to re-establish nutrient and moisture concentrations. Organic produce, although often higher in nutritional value and without direct pesticide exposure, is still subjected to the same environmental factors.

Once food is purchased and taken home, it is often fried, boiled, baked, or microwaved. Most cooking methods result in a loss of nutrients, especially water soluble nutrients like vitamin C and betacarotene[5]. Microwaving is a controversial issue; it may preserve some nutrients more than other cooking methods, but radiation is not a natural way to prepare a meal. Overall, from the time when the food is picked to when it reaches your dinner plate, the nutrient value can be significantly depleted.

Then comes the food processing industry. This industry was developed to extend the shelf life of food, increase food safety and reduce contamination, improve taste, and cater to the ever increasing demands from modern society for immediate, tasty food that is quick to prepare. The processing of food has many advantages, but in terms of nutritional importance, has many disadvantages. This is because during the processing of food, certain nutritious components of the food are often removed. Sometimes synthetic nutrients are added back in, but the food does not resemble its natural and original form which was perfectly designed by nature.

Artificial additives are often added to improve taste, texture, or shelf life. Artificial additives are something that the body does not recognise or have a use for. They are regarded as a foreign substance by the body and therefore, energy and nutrients are employed to aid in their removal. This takes nutrients and energy away from other important physiological processes.

Based on this information, I'm sure you can see that due to modern farming and food processing, our nutrient intake from even a balanced healthy diet may not be enough for our bodies. Add to this the increased 'demands' for nutrients by people in the fast paced, stressful, and toxic life of modern society, and you have a society of people who are missing out on *optimal* amounts of essential nutrients. And because nutrients are what keep our bodies working well, when we don't get enough, we don't 'work' as well as we should.

b) Environmental toxins and external stressors:

We are living in a chemical world. Since the 20th century, about 75,000 chemicals have been introduced into society[6]. We have been bombarded with toxins and have not had time to adjust or adapt to the onslaught. So what is a toxin? In a general sense, it is a substance that is foreign to the body that can either damage tissue or interfere with bodily functions. Some toxins can also be produced in the body as a byproduct of metabolism, and then eliminated via organs such as the liver and kidneys. In this instance however, we are talking about environmental toxins.

Environmental toxins can be found in the air (pollution), on foods, in carpets, cars, household cleaning products, skin care and cosmetic products, in plastics, clothing, on furniture, and even in our non-stick cookware. Electromagnetic radiation can also be considered a toxin, coming from your computer, mobile/cell phones, and microwave oven.

Don't we have organs in the body that get rid of toxins? Yes we do, however, we are living in a world of toxic overload, where we are taking in more chemicals and producing more toxic byproducts than we can handle. This, combined with the fact that we are deficient in many nutrients required for proper detoxification, our bodies are struggling to adapt. As a naturopath, I see many people whose health improves simply by reducing their toxic load and by enhancing the function of their elimination organs. It is worthy to note here that standard blood tests such as liver function tests will only pick up problems that have progressed to a more severe state, or damage that has occurred, they won't necessarily pick up how well your liver is 'functioning', despite the name.

So how do toxins cause or contribute to disease? Well, because they interfere with the normal structure and function of our cells, they disrupt the state of balance. They may enhance some processes, and inhibit others. They may bind to certain nutrients rendering them unavailable, or impair their absorption from the intestinal tract. Some toxins, such as asbestos, cause specific diseases (asbestosis and mesothelioma), and others create non-specific effects which may affect multiple organs systems.

Any chemical that has endocrine (hormonal) disrupting effects such as oestrogen mimicking activity, can be called a 'xenoestrogen'. These oestrogens are from outside the body. Oestrogens produced inside the body are called 'endogenous oestrogens'.

Parabens are a group of toxins that almost everyone is exposed to from skin care, cosmetic products, and sunscreens. They act as a preservative to give the product a longer shelf life, but unfortunately, they have been linked to certain health problems. These chemicals are easily absorbed through the skin into the bloodstream, and can act as endocrine disrupting agents. Even though they are added to many anti-ageing skin care creams, they actually speed up ageing of the skin by increasing the damaging process of 'lipid oxidation' when exposed to ultraviolet light[7]. There have also been some reports of parabens being found in breast cancer tissue[8]. Whether this has any direct relationship on the cancer development is yet to be confirmed.

Some other common chemicals we are exposed to in a low grade accumulative way are:

- **Bisphenol-A:**

This is a chemical with oestrogen-mimicking effects, another endocrine disrupting agent. It is found in plastics, especially those that are softer, eg: water bottles, fast food containers. If this chemical makes its way into the body, it disrupts beta cell function in the pancreas, the gland that produces insulin, and induces insulin resistance. There are also other 'plasticisers' in plastic products that have harmful effects as well.

- **Sodium laureth sulfate:**

This chemical acts as a surfactant or detergent, it is the thing that allows products to foam or froth. It is used in cleaning products, shampoo, toothpaste, and facial cleansers, and may cause skin irritations and the formation of other toxic byproducts.

- **Formaldehyde:**

A possible human carcinogen (cancer-causing chemical), it is a gas that can be found in nail polish, bubble bath and liquid soaps, deodorants, and other products. Because it is a gas, it tends to cause effects within the nose and respiratory system.

It may also cause other systemic effects affecting the reproductive and nervous system.

- **Teflon:**

This product contains various chemicals that make cookware non-stick. The chemicals are released during heating, and have been found in people's bloodstreams and even in mother's breast milk.

These are just a few examples of the many toxins we are exposed to. Some authorities say that chemicals such as these are safe because we aren't exposed to high amounts, but you need to be aware that most of us are exposed to these sorts of chemicals in small but regular 'doses', and an accumulative effect may occur. Also, there is no way to study what effect all these combinations of toxins are having on our bodies. Considering there are over 75,000 chemicals in our environment, how can we possibly be sure of the safety of the trillions of possible combinations that we are exposed to? It makes good sense to reduce our exposure as much as possible, and take steps to maximize our health and ability to detoxify our body.

c) Perceived stress and negative thought patterns:

We all know that stress can have negative effects on your health, but stress is a bit of an overused and general term. What we are talking about really is our perception and reaction to what's going on around us. Some people perceive things as more threatening than they really are, and this depends a lot on our conditioning, the way we are brought up. Some might say it is also due to your genes, which may be true to a certain extent, but the reality is that your perception has more of an effect on your genes than your genes do on your perception!

Let me explain... Your genes are like an instruction manual. They contain the information needed to create something, in this case, your cells, tissues, organs, hormones, and other molecules. Genes do not *control* your body, they are simply the blueprint that houses your 'potential'.

Think of this analogy... You have a list of instructions for putting together say, a piece of furniture. The instructions don't make the furniture, the person reading them does. Even though the instructions have all the information that can create the furniture, it relies on outside intervention to achieve its aim. And depending on the person (or the type of outside influence), the furniture may be put together in several different ways, based on the interpretation of the instructions. The furniture may be put together perfectly, the way it was designed, or the wrong type of screw may be put in the wrong spot, some tools may be missing and therefore the construction is not as strong as it should be. Many things can go wrong, depending on the outside influences.

It is the same with your genes. If the outside influences are positive and appropriate, your genes will produce the highest quality 'version' of you, if the outside influences are negative or there are missing 'tools' such as nutrients, certain genes may be activated while others are inhibited, and abnormal genes or genes for undesirable characteristics may be expressed, creating imbalances in your state of health.

The idea that you can change your state of health by changing your thoughts and perceptions may sound new age and 'out there', but it is in fact rooted in science, discovered by cell biologist Dr Bruce Lipton.

To influence a cell's activity, the cell membrane (outer layer) waits for a signal from its environment. Previously, scientists thought that the genes in the nucleus of the cell controlled the cell's activity, but instead, an outside stimulus controls the genes, and the genes then produce certain effects.

The outside stimulus can be a nutrient, a neurotransmitter, a hormone, or some sort of electrical impulse, energy or vibrational change. We are all made of energy, even apparently inert objects have energy on the atomic level. Thoughts are essentially a vibration, sent throughout our mind and our body. If thoughts are made of energy, and energy can affect a call membrane, then thoughts can affect our cell's activity.

This is a very basic description of what is a complex topic. I recommend reading Dr Lipton's book 'The Biology Of Belief' to gain a greater understanding of one of the most powerful and important discoveries you can use to influence your health in a positive way. If you are a visual learner, I recommend watching one of his DVD's that explains it in an exciting and fun way without feeling like you are in a science lecture!

The main thing to remember is that if your genes affect your health, and your genes are controlled by outside stimuli, then it makes sense to optimize the environment of your cells, by not only getting optimal nutrition and reducing toxic load, but by learning how to change your thoughts and perceptions to ones that will have a positive effect at the cellular level. You will learn ways to do this in section three.

2. Malnourishment, toxic overload, undesirable gene expression.

Examples:

- Nutrient deficiencies
- Nutrient excesses
- Waste build up in digestive tract
- Toxin build up in bloodstream
- Toxin storage in fat cells
- Activation of undesirable genes

2.

a) Malnourishment:

The outcome of poor diet and lifestyle due to poor choices and/or modern farming processes and technology is malnourishment. When we think of the word 'malnourishment', we tend to think of third world countries, but in fact, malnourishment is a very common problem in western countries. Malnourishment means an imbalance of some kind in regards to the body receiving nutrients. People in western countries do not have a deficiency in calories and protein like those in third world countries do, but we have deficiencies or 'sub-optimal intakes' in multiple nutrients, such as certain vitamins, minerals, essential fatty acids, phytochemicals and antioxidants, phytosterols, and glyconutrients. Lower than optimal intake of these nutrients creates a form of malnourishment, putting a stress on our bodies and interfering with normal function. Malnourishment usually relates to deficiencies, but can also mean excesses of certain nutrients, such as carbohydrates or sugars, and sometimes a fat soluble vitamin like vitamin A.

Because we have plenty of food available and a large variety, we think we are getting a balanced diet, and sure we are getting ample calories to provide energy, and protein to build cell structures, the nutrients that keep us alive, but many of us are just not getting enough of the other types of nutrients that modern farming and food processing has depleted from our food supply.

This means that many of us suffer with minor niggling health problems, not realising that many of our symptoms are the body's way of telling us we need a certain nutrient. For example, leg cramps are a common problem for many people, but they are usually attributed to a need for more magnesium. I have not found anyone whose leg cramps have not improved by taking a magnesium supplement. This deficiency is very common, partly due to the fact that there has been a loss of about 21% of magnesium content in fruits and vegetables over a period of thirty years[9]. Magnesium deficiency can also manifest as eye twitches, anxiety, gut pain, period pain, and even high blood pressure. It is also associated with insulin resistance and therefore PCOS. With PCOS, you may also need more chromium and antioxidants.

Sometimes, nutrient deficiencies don't give us any symptoms that we can notice, but instead cause gradual changes inside our bodies that we don't know anything about until the problem gets much worse. For example, a deficiency in essential fatty acids can lead to your cell membranes becoming more rigid and less flexible, making it slightly more difficult for the cell membrane to work properly and allow molecules to enter and exit the cell.

This is something you don't feel or are aware of, so you can't rely on thinking "I feel okay so I must be getting everything from my diet". If you feel okay, that's great, but there may be things going on inside that you are not consciously aware of yet. For example, the most common symptom of heart disease is death. That's right, many people have no early warning, no symptom or sign that anything was wrong until it was too late. Or they may have had slight symptoms and not had them investigated. Symptoms like headaches at the base of the skull, light-headedness, anxiety, gradual weight gain, and not feeling as 'fit' as before. Often symptoms are subtle and people usually attribute them to old age. Just because some symptoms are common does not mean they are normal!

Overall, most people are getting enough nutrients to sustain life, but not enough to sustain a 'quality' of life that is due to optimal health. Optimal health is achieved by receiving adequate amounts of <u>all</u> nutrients.

b) Toxic overload:

As you have already read in Step one, we are living in a toxic world, and our bodies, via evolution, have not fully adapted to this onslaught. It is a daily battle for our elimination organs to deal with toxins entering the body, and our bodies are crying out for help.

Our constant exposure to chemicals puts many of us in a state of toxic overload, whereby we are having to store these chemicals, often in our fat cells, and they are affecting the way our bodies function. I personally believe this toxicity we all face is a major cause of many modern day health complaints, combined with nutritional deficiencies and stress.

c) Undesirable gene expression

The result of negative thoughts and perceptions of stress is 'undesirable gene expression'. What does this mean? First of all, if you have not studied genetics before, you may not realise that all of your genes are not active all of the time. This means that genes are switched on and off, depending on environmental stimulation. Genes are essentially present to provide instructions for building proteins. Proteins make up various components of your body, both structural and functional. The types of proteins made depend on which genes are expressed, and which genes are expressed depends on environmental influences!

Your genes are influenced by your thoughts and perceptions, whether positive or negative. When you break down all the different positive and negative thoughts a person can have, they all boil down to two emotions – love or fear. All negative thoughts are rooted in fear, and positive thoughts rooted in love.

If you are thinking a negative thought, your body is essentially in 'fear' mode, even though you may not feel consciously afraid of anything. What does something do when it is afraid? It hides, attacks, or tries to protect itself. This is exactly what happens in the body with negative perceptions. Genes will be turned on that achieve these aims. You might think protecting itself is a good thing, and it is to a certain extent, but certain disease processes like *inflammation* are in fact a protective mechanism, and it is often the mechanism that in turn creates a problem.

The same goes for hiding. A cell may try to 'hide' from a toxin as best as it can, but because toxins and nutrients usually enter via the same pathways, this means that the cell can also be 'hidden' from the nutrients.

Also, genes may be turned on that activate certain components of the immune system, in an attempt to 'attack' something that you perceived in your environment as a threat. In doing this, it can attack healthy tissue, creating general damage or an autoimmune disease.

On the other hand, what does something or someone do when they feel the emotion of love? They nurture, embrace, and support. This is exactly what happens in the body with positive perceptions. Genes will be turned on that achieve these aims. Your body will be nurtured and supported, and will function in a way that is for your health, wellbeing, and longevity.

Because of the discovery that a cell's environment is what controls the genes, then it goes without saying that to really improve your health you must create an optimal environment to reduce the expression of undesirable genes, and increase the expression of nurturing and supporting genes.

---

3. Abnormal structure, function, communication, & regulation mechanisms in the body.

Examples:
- Excessive cell growth
- Altered chemical reactions/impaired metabolism
- Reduced hormone receptors
- Malfunctioning hormone receptors
- Low pH
- Impaired defence against free radicals
- Toxin binding to receptors
- Antagonism of nutrients by toxins
- Bowel dysbiosis
- Increased intestinal permeability (leaky gut syndrome)
- Altered glycoprotein formation
- Miscommunication between cells

3.

a) Abnormal cell structure, function, communication, and regulation:

The main result of malnourishment, toxic overload, and undesirable gene expression is simply that the body fails to work properly. Some symptoms may appear at this stage, but many don't.

With a deficiency of essential fatty acids combined with eating or producing too much cholesterol, cell membranes can become more rigid. This makes it hard for nutrients and molecules to enter or leave the cell, and it also makes arteries and other blood vessels less flexible and less able to deal with pressure changes. If affecting your red blood cells, they may be less able to squeeze in and out of capillaries to deliver oxygen, resulting in cold extremities, and possibly fatigue.

Malnourishment involving an 'excess' of things such as carbohydrates or sugars can result in your body storing excess energy in fat cells. This creates an imbalance in body composition, with more fat and less muscle. Low protein intakes, especially on weight loss diets, can result in a breakdown of protein from your own cells like muscle cells, reducing the amount of active metabolic tissue available for energy production.

The number and structure of cell membrane receptors can be affected by malnourishment and expression of certain genes. If receptor numbers are reduced, the hormone they are made for will have less of an effect, and over time the hormone secretion may be increased, in an attempt to produce more receptors to deal with the demand. This is what can happen in the development of insulin resistance. If receptors are malformed due to missing nutrients, toxic damage, or certain genes, they may not function normally, and the hormone may not be able to bind to the receptor, or may only bind weakly, producing less of the hormone's desired effects. If abnormal, they may also allow binding of other molecules that happen to fit the receptor better, messing up hormonal balance.

When you are deficient in certain nutrients, some aspects of your metabolism may not work properly. For example, we need B vitamins to extract energy from carbohydrate foods. A high intake of carbohydrates tends to use up a lot of B vitamins, making energy production from food less efficient. Alcohol also uses up B vitamins, especially vitamin B1 (thiamin). This deficiency can make you crave carbohydrates even more. Because you are not extracting as much energy from the food, the body tries to rectify the problem by getting you to eat more 'energy' in the form of food.

Cell to cell communication is another important process in the body that can be affected by malnourishment. Every day, your cells are communicating with each other. They are 'saying' things like "Nourish me, I need some vitamin C", or "Regulate me, I need more or less of this hormone", or "Don't attack me, I am one of you".

Cellular communication requires molecules such as glyconutrients, which are reduced in the modern diet. So how do cells communicate? They communicate mostly via glycoprotein structures on cell membranes. These glycoproteins have various functions, one of which is to allow the immune system to recognise whether a certain cell is part of the body or whether it is foreign to the body, and therefore whether to attack it or not. If this process is hampered by malformed glycoproteins, the immune system may not be able to recognize the cell and may attack it anyway (an autoimmune disease).

Glycoproteins are made of protein and carbohydrates. The carbohydrate components are not the same as the sugar you eat in foods. There are actually seven other types of carbohydrates in addition to sugar that are called 'glyconutrients'. Glyconutrients are molecules that form structures in the body such as glycoproteins. They are the vital parts of the glycoprotein that allows cells to communicate with each other. If any glyconutrients are missing or deficient, the glycoprotein will not form correctly and cell communication will be impaired or altered.

Glyconutrients are found mostly in foods such as gums, saps, algae, aloe vera, some herbs, and some vegetables, but they usually develop in plants the final stages of vine ripening. Because green harvesting interrupts this process, modern food is deficient in most of the glyconutrients that are necessary for cell communication. Five of the eight glyconutrients are also found in breast milk, illustrating the important role they play in human health. The body can make glyconutrients to a certain extent, but this takes time, energy, and multiple enzymatic steps requiring other nutrients. If any nutrients required are in short supply, this process will be slow or impaired. Also, specific transporters for some of these glyconutrients have been found in the gastrointestinal tract, indicating that the body prefers to get them from a dietary source.

Because we are not getting an adequate intake of glyconutrients today, many people suffer with symptoms that result from miscommunication in the body. As you know, a breakdown in communication can affect many aspects of your life, your work, your family, your partnerships, and your friendships. It is the same in the human body, a lack of harmony results, causing a variety of problems.

A good analogy to understand the important role glyconutrients play in communication is with email addresses. If you get one letter wrong, or miss one out, the intended recipient won't get the message, or the wrong person may get the message. The same goes for our cells. If a glycoprotein has missing or deficient glyconutrients, the cellular message won't get delivered to where it needs to go, or it might get sent somewhere else, causing malfunction in the body. More will be discussed about glyconutrients as they relate to your health, in section three.

Malnourishment and toxic overload also affects your pH balance. Your pH determines how acidic or alkaline your body is. A simple urine test can determine your pH. It should be around 7.0. Anything under about 6.5 and your body is too acidic.

Regulation of pH occurs naturally in a healthy body. If you are too acidic it means that your body is not able to regulate or eliminate the excess acidic waste as effectively as it should. Modern diets, high intake of processed foods and carbonated beverages, combined with toxin exposure, create a lot of acidic waste products in the body. Achieving and maintaining normal pH becomes a struggle for many people; most are unaware of the problem. When pH is abnormal, certain enzymes won't work properly, meaning that some chemical reactions will be impaired, affecting the body's metabolism.

Also, with a low pH, calcium can be taken from tissues such as bone and sent to the bloodstream to 'buffer' the acid, raising the pH. When this occurs excessively, bone calcium levels can become low, making bones weaker, and the high blood calcium can lead to complications such as calcium deposits in joints and arteries.

A low pH in the tissues can also result in fluid retention. This is because water is a natural way of diluting the acid. If you spilled some kind of strong acid on your skin, what would you do? You would run it under water. The same happens in the body.

Abnormal regulation mechanisms can also result in abnormal growth and development of cells. Cells may fail to reproduce or develop adequately, or they may reproduce too quickly and multiply rapidly (as in tumours). Cysts in the ovaries (follicular cysts) develop because of a lack of ovulation, which prevents the follicle from maturing and developing into the corpus luteum. This is due to both abnormal regulation mechanisms and miscommunication between cells.

Malnourishment combined with toxic overload can also result in a deficiency of antioxidants. Antioxidants protect our cells from free radicals, molecules produced with daily metabolism that disrupt the structure of our cells, damaging them and contributing to cell malfunction and the ageing process. Antioxidants help prevent free radicals from 'attacking' our cells.

One of the common consequences of the world we live in is the development of what we call 'bowel dysbiosis'. This is an imbalance between the levels of good and bad bacteria in the digestive tract. Normally the digestive tract contains various types of bacteria that are beneficial for our immune systems, our digestive systems, and for production of some nutrients. In a healthy bowel, the 'good' bugs should outnumber the 'bad' bugs, but in most people today, the bad bugs predominate. Poor diets, alcohol, stress, and some medications like the contraceptive pill and antibiotics disrupt the normal balance. This then creates problems with digestion, immune function, and nutrient production, and can cause inflammation and increased intestinal permeability (what naturopaths call 'leaky gut syndrome').

Leaky gut basically means that the space between the cells lining the digestive tract becomes larger, allowing larger molecules into the bloodstream. These larger molecules can be undigested food proteins, bacteria, parasites, and fungi. This can set off many inflammatory and allergic reactions in the bloodstream.

Figure 3

a) **Normal digestive tract:**

b) **'Leaky' digestive tract:**

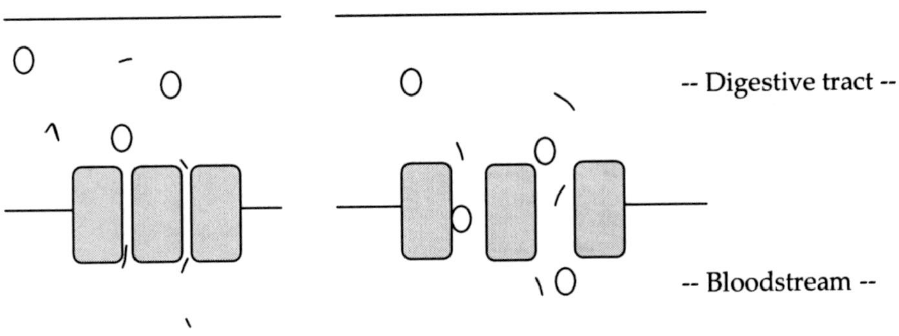

-- Digestive tract --

-- Bloodstream --

a) Larger molecules (e.g.: undigested food) cannot pass through the tight junctions between intestinal cells in the gut wall.

b) Larger molecules *can* pass through the junctions between intestinal cells because the gut wall has become more permeable due to toxins, bacterial overgrowth and inflammation, stress hormones, alcohol.

4. Abnormal manifestations, undesirable adaptive and compensatory mechanisms.

Examples:

- Insulin resistance
- Increased inflammation
- Impaired fat metabolism
- Hormonal imbalances
- Oxidative stress
- High blood pressure
- Neurotransmitter imbalances
- Impaired cellular energy production
- Autoimmune processes
- Poor immune function & susceptibility to infections
- Over-reactivity, allergic reactions

4.

a) Abnormal manifestations, undesirable adaptive and compensatory mechanisms:

At this stage of disease progression, measurable changes can often be detected by lab tests, and certain signs may be picked up by medical examination. The abnormal structure, function, communication, and regulation mechanisms outlined in step three result in these manifestations.

Insulin resistance and hyperinsulinaemia, where the body produces more insulin in an attempt to get glucose (sugar) from the bloodstream into the cells, results from impaired regulation, communication, function, and sometimes impaired receptor structure (step three). As you know, these impairments are caused by the previous step, malnourishment, toxic overload, and undesirable gene expression (step two). Can you see how this is all starting to fit together?

Due to impaired regulation and communication mechanisms, inflammation may be increased, fat metabolism is hampered, and hormones and neurotransmitters become imbalanced (e.g.: high testosterone, high LH, low serotonin, high cortisol).

Oxidative stress results from the excess free radicals, due to a deficiency of antioxidants. Oxidative stress is when the amount of free radicals overwhelms the body's antioxidant defense mechanisms, creating damage to cell structure and function, and even DNA. Women with PCOS often have increased oxidative stress, and this can contribute to an increased risk of cardiovascular disease[10].

High blood pressure is an example of a manifestation due to abnormal structure, function, regulation, and communication. It is not a symptom as you cannot 'feel' it or 'see' it, and it is not a disease, it is a sign of underlying imbalances. It may result from arteries being too stiff or going into spasm (structure and function), abnormal hormone secretion (regulation), or impaired feedback to the brain (communication). Or it can simply be an adaptive mechanism due to excess weight gain, increasing the blood pressure in an attempt to deliver nutrients and oxygen further from the heart to the excess amount of body tissue.

Impaired cellular communication and leaky gut syndrome may lead to immune system dysregulation, resulting in things such as tissue damage from an autoimmune process, increased markers in the blood that indicate an allergic process, and poor immune defense resulting in an increased likelihood of infections.

These are just a few examples of the many manifestations that can occur due to the disease progression process. You will also see in figure two that step three and four tend to occur in a cycle, a vicious cycle. Many of the occurrences in these two steps overlap, and they tend to exacerbate each other. For example, reduced receptors (step 3) can contribute to insulin resistance (step 4), and insulin resistance can cause further reduction in receptors. Also, increased gut permeability (step 3) can cause inflammatory reactions in the body (step 4), and inflammatory reactions can cause a further increase in gut permeability!

---

5. Noticeable symptoms.

Examples:

- Weight gain/obesity
- Acne
- Hair loss
- Excess body hair
- Irregular menstrual cycles
- Sweet cravings, excess hunger
- Depression and anxiety
- Constipation and diarrhoea
- Fatigue
- Headaches & migraines
- Muscle and joint aches

5.

a) Noticeable symptoms:

Symptoms are the noticeable manifestations of the underlying imbalances we have discussed. They are the outward effects of health in crisis. They are not the first indication of disease, but in fact a 'last chance cry for help' from the body, as a way of saying "Things are out of balance in here – do something!"

Sweet cravings or a strong desire for carbohydrate foods like bread, pasta, candy, cakes, etc, is a symptom. It is the body's way of saying "I need more energy and I want to feel good". But if you look deeper it is really saying "My cells are not getting enough sugar for energy production because my insulin is not working properly at getting sugar inside the cells". Therefore, eating sugar may give you some temporary benefit, but you are still not fixing the cause of the problem.

Irregular menstrual cycles are a symptom, something you can notice, especially if you are trying to conceive. The body is trying to say "My hormones are not in balance; this is not the most conducive environment for a baby to develop, please regulate me". You have the choice of artificially creating a hormonal environment conducive to conception, or the choice of looking at why the environment is not conducive, and taking steps to fix the underlying problems naturally.

People with the same disease can vary in the types of symptoms they experience. This is because of the variation in all the underlying causes in step one to four. Also, two people with the same symptom may find that the triggers that allow development of that symptom might be slightly different. For example, someone might have acne that is mostly due to bowel dysbiosis and the resulting toxicity and inflammation, whereas, another person with acne might also have some degree of this, but their main issue might be one of negative perception about their physical appearance, resulting in undesirable gene expression affecting their skin's response to hormonal stimulation.

Can you see how your symptoms are a message from the inside, alerting you to the imbalances that lie within? What is your body trying to tell you?

---

6. Diagnosis and classification of a disease name.

Examples:

- Polycystic ovary syndrome
- Irritable bowel syndrome
- Chronic fatigue syndrome
- Pre-diabetes
- Hypothyroidism
- Arthritis
- Asthma
- Generalised anxiety disorder
- Clinical depression

6.

a) Diagnosis and classification of a disease name:

Step six is when you are officially diagnosed as having a 'disease'. Diagnosis usually results from a combination of test results, your symptoms, and your family history.

Certain symptoms when they present together, can be classified as a certain disease. Symptoms are like ingredients in a recipe for disease. The type of disease you have depends on the combination of symptoms. Just like the type of meal you are making depends on the combination of ingredients. The ingredients are not always exclusive to that meal; some may be combined with other ingredients to make a completely different meal. In the same way, many symptoms are not exclusive to a certain disease; they can be combined with other symptoms to create another different disease.

For example, you may suffer with irregular periods, acne, fatigue, weight gain, and hair loss, and be diagnosed with PCOS, but you may also be diagnosed with hypothyroidism which can result in some symptoms also occurring in PCOS such as fatigue, weight gain, and hair loss. In addition you may also suffer with constipation and diarrhea, cramping, and bloating, and be diagnosed with irritable bowel syndrome as well. You may also be diagnosed with depression, arthritis, and any number of other diseases, based on whether you have signs or symptoms that are common to that particular disease. Regardless of what disease you have, there are underlying factors that are common amongst all diseases and they need to be addressed to truly get better.

A disease is simply a collection of signs and/or symptoms, brought about by underlying imbalances in cell structure and function, which can be traced back to poor diet and lifestyle, environmental toxins and external stressors, and perceived stress and negative thought patterns.

To help you understand better and put all this information together, I have repeated figure two, this time with some basic examples of factors involved in the development of PCOS. There will be some overlap, some examples will fit into more than one category or step, but this will give you an overview of the big picture of how you developed PCOS.

Figure 4

ORIGINS OF DISEASE
With examples relating to the development of polycystic ovary syndrome

1. Poor diet & lifestyle, environmental toxins and external stressors, negative perceptions & thought patterns.
E.g.: High glycaemic diet & other poor diet choices, processed foods, modern farming practices, little exercise, poor sleep, exposure to xenoestrogens, negative attitude & lack of empowerment about health.

2. Malnourishment, toxic overload, undesirable gene expression.
E.g.: Nutrient deficiencies such as chromium, magnesium, and essential fatty acids. Excess calorie intake, toxins entering body, certain genes activated by environmental factors, thoughts, and perceptions.

4. Abnormal manifestations, undesirable adaptive/compensatory mechanisms.
E.g.: cyst formation, clinical insulin resistance, leptin resistance, high insulin, high testosterone & LH, low progesterone (oestrogen dominance), low grade inflammation, inflammatory/allergic food reactions.

3. Abnormal structure, function, communication, and regulation mechanisms in the body.
E.g.: Anovulation, reduced insulin receptors, malfunctioning insulin receptors and glucose transporters, binding of xenoestrogens to hormone receptors, bowel dysbiosis & increased intestinal permeability.

5. Noticeable symptoms.
E.g.: weight gain, irregular/absent menstrual cycles, carbohydrate cravings & hunger, acne, excess body hair, scalp hair loss, mood swings, fatigue, trouble conceiving.

6. Diagnosis and classification of disease name.

E.g.: Polycystic Ovary Syndrome.

SUMMARY OF HOW PCOS SYMPTOMS MAY DEVELOP

Sometimes it can be easier to understand the initiation and progression of disease if you take a symptom, and go backwards into how it developed. Here we will look at a couple of common PCOS symptoms and trace them back to their possible causes, to give you an idea of how all this relates to you…

Weight gain:

Although not all women with PCOS are overweight, many are. If you are, you may have experienced or be experiencing the frustration of feeling like you are doing everything you are supposed to do to lose weight, but it is just not coming off. The six steps involved in the origin of disease, along with the 7 Step Solution in section three, might give you some insight into what is missing from your approach.

Weight gain, or an inability to lose excess body fat, is a symptom (step 5). It can also be classed as the disease 'obesity' (step 6). Many things can contribute to weight gain, so we will look at some of the most likely causes that relate to weight gain associated with PCOS.

Because you have PCOS, you might have been told your weight gain is due to insulin resistance and that is the cause. But because we know that insulin resistance is part of step 4 in disease progression, we know it is not the root cause.

So we take a step back and ask "what is causing the insulin resistance which is causing me to gain weight?". It may be that you don't have enough insulin receptors, or your receptors are malformed, or your glucose transporters (molecules that travel to the cell membrane to 'pick up' glucose from the blood) are faulty or damaged, or there are not enough of them. One or all of these factors (step 3) may be underlying your insulin resistance.

But why don't you have enough receptors? Or why are your receptors or glucose transporters damaged and not working properly? It may be due to a manifestation such as inflammation in step 4 (the vicious cycle is occurring) that is damaging them, and/or it may be due to an excess of carbohydrates entering the bloodstream, chromium and magnesium deficiency, or activation of genes that produce abnormal insulin receptors (step 2).

We know that excess carbohydrates entering the bloodstream is due to a combination of eating too many carbohydrate containing foods, and also eating foods that have a high glycaemic index which allows carbohydrates to be absorbed into the bloodstream more quickly. We also know that chromium and magnesium deficiency may result from a combination of not eating foods high in these nutrients, or simply from modern farming practices and soil depletion that is preventing you from getting enough in your diet, even if you are eating a balanced diet. In addition to this, we also know that the abnormal genes (in this example, for the insulin receptor), are activated by a cell's environment which depends on nutrient concentrations, toxins, and most importantly, your perceptions, attitudes, and beliefs (step1).

So from the symptom of weight gain, we have travelled from step 5 back to step 1, and you can see where your 'treatment' *should* be targeted.

Excess facial and body hair:

One of the most distressing and de-feminising symptoms of PCOS, hirsutism can vary from mild and hardly noticeable, to severe and needing removal every day.

Hirsutism is a symptom (step 5). Taking a step back, we discover that it is usually due to high testosterone (step 4). High testosterone can be due to insulin resistance (insulin increases testosterone), low sex hormone binding globulin (SHBG), or higher conversion of testosterone precursors in the skin and hair cells (still step 4).

Collectively, these factors can be caused by insufficient or faulty insulin receptors and glucose transporters, having too much body fat and not enough lean muscle tissue, and possibly your skin cells and hair follicles are genetically more 'sensitive' to testosterone (step 3). Also, you will see in a moment that not having enough good bacteria in the digestive tract can make you low in SHBG (SHBG binds hormones like testosterone, making it unable to affect the skin and hair).

Going back even further you might find that the increased sensitivity to testosterone, the poor body composition (too much fat, not enough muscle), and the faulty or deficient insulin receptors and glucose transporters are due to a high glycaemic diet, chromium and magnesium deficiencies, and/or undesirable gene expression (step 2). You may also be deficient in soluble fibre intake (needed to stimulate SHBG, via fermentation by gut bacteria), which means that your SHBG production is lower, and therefore the amount of testosterone affecting your skin is higher.

Again we come back to step 1, poor diet choices, modern farming practices, and soil depletion causing the high exposure to carbohydrates, and the deficiency of nutrients like chromium, magnesium, and fibre. There is also the toxin exposure causing wide ranging problems with hormones and upsetting the balance of gut bacteria, and negative perceptions and thoughts causing undesirable gene expression (such as those controlling testosterone sensitivity).

Can you see that regardless of whether you are most concerned with weight gain or excess hair, you need to focus on exactly the same starting point? So instead of finding a 'treatment' for each different symptom, why not start at the beginning and get positive results with ALL symptoms.

IS YOUR TREATMENT TARGETING THE CAUSES OF PCOS?

Here you will find out which of the six steps your current treatments are targeted at. Although you may be undergoing some treatments or therapies that aren't listed here, this discussion is to give you a basic idea of where each general treatment works within your body.

Surgery:

Surgery such as ovarian drilling (to remove cysts/follicles and excess tissue that is secreting testosterone), can improve symptoms for some women. It is targeting step five, a symptom. Although it is removing existing cysts, and some follicles that may be on their way to forming a cyst, it is not removing the cause or the tendency for cysts to be formed.

Hysterectomy, the removal of the uterus with or without removal of the ovaries, is a radical and irreversible procedure to get rid of severe menstrual related problems like ongoing bleeding, severe pain...etc. It will cause an artificial menopause, and if the ovaries are removed, a huge reduction in hormones such as oestrogen and testosterone. However, certain other cells in the body can produce these hormones. (such as fat cells and the adrenal glands).

A hysterectomy will target step five, the symptoms, but it may also target step four and step three because it is physically removing the organs that some of the abnormal structure, function, and manifestations are associated with. A hysterectomy will not 'cure' your PCOS or deal with the underlying causes though, as it is not purely a reproductive problem, but a metabolic problem affecting the whole body.

Drugs:

A medication such as metformin acts at step four and possibly step three. It is helping to reduce insulin secretion and also making your cells more 'sensitive' to insulin, thereby targeting insulin resistance, a manifestation. Although insulin resistance is not the root cause, it is a major driver for your symptoms. Targeting insulin resistance directly, as well as dealing with the underlying causes at step one and two, is a good combination to help you achieve quicker and better results. As you will see in section three, there are several solutions for targeting insulin resistance naturally.

Fertility drugs such as clomid, work at step three, by encouraging ovulation. If you are not ovulating and you take clomid, it may help you ovulate and therefore increase the possibility of conceiving. It is not targeting the exact cause of the lack of ovulation though; it is actually working at the vicious cycle between step three and four, impacting the hormonal manifestations at step four, to encourage ovulation at step three. With a *lack* of ovulation comes the hormonal imbalances at step four and with the hormonal imbalances comes more problems with ovulating.

Other fertility treatments such as follicle stimulating hormone (FSH) injections, target step four, increasing FSH to stimulate development of the ovarian follicle which may lead to ovulation.

The contraceptive or birth control pill is a drug containing synthetic hormones. It creates an artificial cycle and induces regular periods, while preventing ovulation from occurring. It targets step four, the manifestations, by changing the hormonal profile of the patient to one that reduces symptoms such as acne, excess hair, and irregular cycles. Contrary to popular belief, the pill does NOT 'regulate' your cycle. It gives you an artificial cycle, masking some of the symptoms of PCOS. Although it can reduce some symptoms, most pills actually make insulin resistance worse, and they also contribute to bowel dysbiosis (step three), two of the underlying factors involved in PCOS!

Although drugs are treating your symptoms and can bring relief, keep in mind that they are also contributing to one of the underlying causes of PCOS - toxic overload. Remember, all drugs are toxins by classification, which is the reason they have side effects.

Herbs:

Herbs are plants, many of which have medicinal or therapeutic benefit. Many drugs are based on an active ingredient in a plant, isolated and reproduced synthetically. Herbs when used for health conditions are called herbal medicines. There are wide varieties of herbs that can work on certain areas of the body, either individually or in a synergistic combination with other herbs.

As a naturopath you may expect me to say that herbs work at the underlying causes, but this is not completely true. Depending on which particular herb you are talking about, herbs work at several of the steps in disease progression. Like drugs, they work at step three, affecting abnormal functions and regulation mechanisms, to bring about a reduction in the manifestations which can lead to symptoms. Some also work at step two, providing nutrients to the body to enable it to function better, and reducing toxic overload by increasing your body's ability to detoxify itself.

Also, some herbs may affect step one indirectly, by working at step three and four - improving the hormones and regulation mechanisms involved with balancing your mood, therefore making it easier for you to change your perceptions and thoughts to more positive ones.

Herbs can be very useful, and many have physiological effects comparable to that of medications. An example is St John's Wort, in relation to the treatment of depression. Herbs should not be used on their own in the treatment of PCOS, because they are not targeting all triggers and causes. The body is not deficient in herbs, as it is not deficient in drugs, and so you must look first at what the body *needs*.

Diet changes & nutritional supplements:

Improving your diet directly affects step one, and can have great effects on your health. Making better choices allows you to reduce malnourishment, by receiving a higher amount of necessary nutrients, and preventing an excessive intake of certain nutrients, unhealthy diet components, and toxins.

Eating a healthy balanced diet is always the first step to take in improving your health, regardless of the condition you have, however, there are certain dietary modifications that are more suitable for specific conditions. (for example, a low glycaemic index diet for diabetics and women with PCOS, or a low protein diet for those with kidney disease…etc).

Even if you eat a healthy diet, as you will have learned, our modern way of farming and living has reduced our intake of many nutrients. Nutritional supplements deal with the gap between what nature provides, and what we actually get, providing you with an optimal intake of nutrients to allow your body to function better. Therefore, they target step one and two, reducing the effects on our bodies from modern farming practices, and providing us with optimal nutrient intake to prevent malnourishment. Certain nutrients are also more important for certain conditions, not directly, but by being used up more quickly as part of the process of that disease, or via genetic factors that make an individual more susceptible to a certain deficiency. You will learn in section three which nutritional supplements are essential for overall health, and which may have therapeutic benefit for PCOS.

Exercise:

Exercise is not really a treatment as such, but a natural activity that human beings are designed for, and activity that maintains our health, but can also have specific and significant effects on people with certain conditions such as PCOS.

Exercise targets step one in a couple of ways. It helps form part of a healthy lifestyle, and it can also influence the expression of certain genes which have a beneficial role in the body. Through these effects, exercise can improve many symptoms of PCOS, for example, by making your cells more sensitive to insulin, and by increasing your metabolic rate to help you lose excess body fat.

Psychological and mind-body therapies:

Taking care of your psychological health, and participating in specific techniques and therapies that change your thought patterns target step one. By changing your thought patterns, they can directly affect which genes are 'switched on' and which ones are 'turned off'. Therefore, part of any treatment should include strategies to deal with negative perceptions, to prevent or reduce the expression of undesirable genes.

Figure 5: How treatments intervene in the disease process

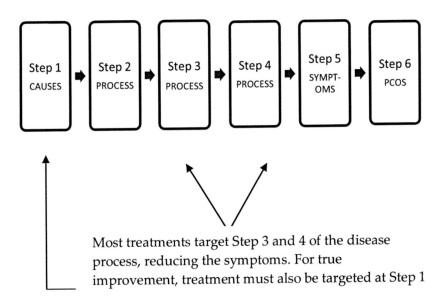

Most treatments target Step 3 and 4 of the disease process, reducing the symptoms. For true improvement, treatment must also be targeted at Step 1

Some of you might be thinking… "I already eat a healthy diet, I take a multivitamin, I exercise, and I try to maintain a positive attitude. Why aren't I getting better?". There is another factor involved in step one - exposure to environmental toxins that MUST be dealt with in order to REALLY improve.

Also, you may believe you have a positive attitude, but there is a lot more to changing your thought patterns, and therefore reducing undesirable gene expression, than just being positive. Certain things must be done 'deliberately' each day to maximise this power we all have.

Although I got a reduction in my own symptoms by using many different treatments and therapies, I didn't achieve complete success until I targeted both detoxification, and the power of the mind. Section three will tell you things you must do to achieve success, and things you can do additionally if you choose, to improve your results even more.

Let's get started!!

SECTION THREE

SOLUTIONS

*Empowering yourself and
regaining balance*

In order to get results and achieve success, there are various steps that must be taken. There is no 'magic pill' or 'one treatment' that is going to allow you to achieve success over polycystic ovary syndrome. It is a condition with many underlying factors, and requires a combination of strategies to be utilised.

I have developed a 7 Step Solution for you to follow; it targets both the symptoms and the causes of PCOS, and gets right at step one in the disease progression model discussed in the previous section. **If poor diet and lifestyle, environmental toxins and stressors, and negative perceptions and thought patterns are the most basic triggers/causes of PCOS, then the solutions *must* counteract these problems. The solutions must encompass nourishment, protection, and positivity.**

Nourishment counteracts a poor diet and lifestyle, preventing malnourishment. Protection counteracts the toxins and stressors, preventing toxic overload, and Positivity counteracts the negative perceptions, preventing undesirable gene expression. By targeting these three things, we have interrupted the progression to step two, and therefore step three and so on. Could it really be this simple?

Figure 6:   Three Simple Steps To Health

~~Poor diet & lifestyle,~~ 1. NOURISHMENT ~~environmental toxins and~~ ~~external stressors,~~ 2. PROTECTION ~~negative perceptions &~~ ~~thought patterns.~~ 3. POSITIVITY	HEALTH 1. The body receives optimal nutrition. 2. Toxins are reduced, neutralised and eliminated. 3. Healthy genes are expressed.

Okay, now let's get down to business. So you have been diagnosed with PCOS or you suspect you have PCOS, what do you do now? First you must 'assess' where you are at, to know where you want to be. Then you must prioritise your success plan, depending on your individual needs. The following diagram allows you to see the big picture of what you need to do.

Figure 7: What to do after a diagnosis of PCOS

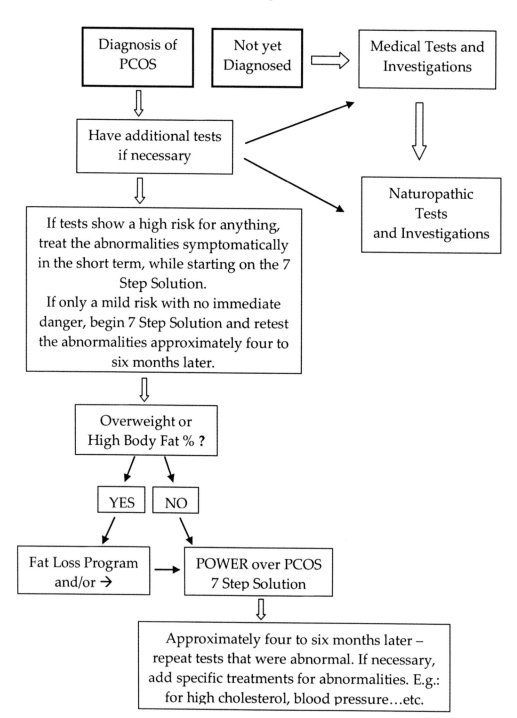

ASSESSING YOUR STATE OF HEALTH:

Assessing your state of health can involve both self assessment via observations and questionnaires, and testing procedures arranged through a health professional.

If you are not sure whether you have PCOS, you would need to see a doctor or specialist (usually an endocrinologist or gynaecologist) to confirm the diagnosis and rule out any other conditions. If you are reading this book you most likely already know you have PCOS. I suggest keeping a file with records of all your medical appointments and their outcomes, and asking for copies of all test results so you can keep track of your own state of health.

If you have already had a variety of tests, check the following list to see if there's anything else you would like to discuss with your health professional, to determine which tests would be beneficial in finding out more about where your health is at, and pinpointing any specific problem areas. You may also wish to explore some of the naturopathic tests available through certain practitioners, some of which I find extremely useful to discover underlying imbalances, and also to monitor your progress and keep you motivated.

Medical tests:

- Medical history, symptom evaluation, and physical examination

- Glucose tolerance test (GTT) with fasting, one hour, and two hour insulin levels.

- Insulin must be tested as well as glucose. A normal glucose level does not rule out insulin resistance.

- SHBG, FAI, Testosterone.

These stand for sex hormone binding globulin and free androgen index. SHBG can be low in PCOS, which can make the FAI high. Basically this means that more hormone is available to act on your tissues.

- Oestrogen and progesterone.

If you not experiencing amenorrhea (lack of periods), it is ideal to measure these hormones in the second half of the cycle.

- LH and FSH.

Luteinising hormone and follicle stimulating hormone. LH surges before ovulation, but can be sustained at a high level in some women with PCOS. FSH stimulates development of the follicles in the ovaries. Sometimes, but not always, the LH to FSH ratio is high.

- Prolactin.

Prolactin normally encourages breast milk production. In some non-pregnant and non-lactating women with PCOS, it is abnormally high. This can be due to stress, excessive exercise, certain medications, low dopamine levels, or a prolactin secreting tumour of the pituitary gland.

- TSH.

Testing for thyroid stimulating hormone determines whether your thyroid gland may be under or over functioning. Thyroid hormones may be tested as well. When your thyroid is underactive, TSH levels will usually be high (because it is trying to 'stimulate' the gland to function). When your thyroid gland is overactive, the TSH will be low.

- Fasting lipid studies, HDL, and LDL.

These will assess various fats and cholesterol levels in the blood. Triglycerides and LDL can sometimes be high in PCOS. HDL is high density lipoprotein and caries excess cholesterol away from cells for elimination, LDL is low density lipoprotein and delivers cholesterol to the cells.

- hsCRP.

C-Reactive protein is a protein produced by the liver and is a sign of inflammation. It can be used as a general assessment tool, and is sometimes used to assess your risk for heart disease.

- Homocysteine.

An intermediate compound in protein metabolism. If it accumulates it can become a risk factor for atherosclerosis, and therefore heart disease. Some studies have shown it to be high in women with PCOS, especially those with insulin resistance.

- Full blood count and general biochemistry.

An FBC or CBC is often routinely done when ordering blood tests. It gives an overall idea of the health of your blood cells and immune system.

- LFT.

Liver function test. This picks up raised liver enzymes which are indicative of damage to the liver or some underlying pathology. Technically, it is not a 'liver function test' but more of a 'liver damage test'.

- Blood pressure.

A non-invasive and easy test to determine the pressure exerted by your blood against the blood vessels, during both contraction and relaxation of the heart muscle. Ideal BP is approximately 110/70 to 120/80. The first number is the pressure when the heart is contracting (systolic), the second number is when the heart is relaxing (diastolic) before the next beat. Systolic can fluctuate more than diastolic, especially in response to stress or exercise.

- Pelvic ultrasound.

This test is used to view the uterus and ovaries, and determine the presence of cysts. This test can be useful when confirming a diagnosis of PCOS, but is not essential.

- Coeliac screening.

If you are having trouble conceiving, or experience digestive symptoms, chronic low iron levels, or unexplained fatigue, I suggest having a test to rule out coeliac disease, an intolerance to gluten, the protein found in wheat, rye, barley, and some oats. Many cases go undiagnosed for years, and it is worth making sure.

Your doctor may suggest other tests, but those above are the most common.

Naturopathic tests:

- Nutritional/Dietary analysis.

Performed by a naturopath, nutritionist, or dietician. Determines how healthy your diet is, and whether you are likely to be missing out on certain nutrients.

- Lifestyle, exercise, and stress appraisals.

Your lifestyle habits are assessed by a combination of questionnaires and discussion. You may also be referred to a fitness professional for a proper assessment, and you may have additional tests for stress hormones if necessary.

- Total health appraisal.

Naturopaths will assess the function of all your body systems via discussion and often a comprehensive questionnaire. Regardless of what condition you have, the health of your immune, cardiovascular, hormonal, musculoskeletal, liver, digestive, and other systems will be assessed, based on a symptom analysis.

- Body composition.

A body composition test analyses the amount of fat and muscle you have, sometimes also hydration levels and bone mass. It may also determine your metabolic rate and give an approximate guide as to your real biological age. Some naturopaths will have a BIA machine (bioimpedance analyser), also called cellular health analysis, to give an accurate assessment of these biological markers. The test is non-invasive and involves attaching electrodes to specific points on the hands and feet. It is very useful for those wanting to lose weight, as you can monitor your results and make sure you are losing body fat and not muscle tissue.

- Live blood analysis.

In practice I have used Hemaview™ Live Blood Screening. It is a very useful test to get a visual picture of what is going on in your bloodstream. A lancet is used to take a small drop of blood from the fingertip, the blood is then placed under a dark field microscope and analysed while it is still 'alive' and moving around. The image seen through the microscope is projected onto a monitor for the patient to see as well. It is quite amazing and motivating for the patient to see their own blood on the screen.

Live blood analysis is used to determine such things as inflammation, infection, allergy, liver & digestive health, deficiencies or increased demands for essential fatty acids, vitamin B12 and folic acid, how 'sticky' the blood is, platelet aggregations and clotting tendencies, cell damage from mechanical trauma or oxidative stress, increased cell breakdown, cellular dehydration, immune imbalances, and various other specific abnormalities.

Standard blood tests show the 'amounts' of various cells and substances, live blood analysis shows the 'quality' of your blood and immune cells, by looking at the shapes, sizes, variations between cells, movement, and presence of certain substances. It is especially useful to monitor a patient's treatment.

To see some amazing photos that show blood under the microscope before and after treatment, visit:
www.poweroverpcos.com/livebloodanalysis.html

- Zinc tally.

A zinc tally is a taste test to determine the degree of zinc deficiency in a patient. It involves holding a small amount of zinc tally (zinc sulfate heptahydrate – in distilled water) in the mouth for ten seconds, and then swallowing. Zinc status is divided into four categories and depends on how strong the taste is;

1. No taste sensation. Like water.
2. Slight taste develops after a few seconds.
3. A definite, almost immediate taste occurs, and tends to intensify.
4. An immediate, strong, and unpleasant taste.

Category 1 is very low zinc levels, category 4 is optimal zinc levels. Most people are a category 2 when tested, and most people go up to a category 4 after supplementation with liquid zinc. A liquid as opposed to a tablet is needed in a zinc deficient state, because zinc is required for the absorption of zinc! Liquid zinc bypasses the normal absorption route, allowing zinc to be rapidly replenished. Once zinc is replenished, a person can absorb zinc more easily from food and a multivitamin.

- Urine and Saliva pH.

Your pH indicates how acidic or alkaline you are. The optimal pH in urine and saliva samples should be around 7.0. Many people I see in practice have a pH of around 6.0 which is too acidic. A good remedy for this (in addition to proper diet and lifestyle), is freshly squeezed lemon in water a few times a day. This stimulates the release of secretin, a hormone from the small intestine which encourages bicarbonate to be released from the pancreas. This buffers the acid and normalises the pH.

You can arrange to have your pH tested, or you can buy test strips from a pharmacy and test it yourself. Some test strips give a more specific and accurate reading though, so it is worth buying the more expensive ones or doing several tests to get an average reading.

- Oxidative stress test.

There are a few different tests on the market that test for cell damage from free radicals. I assess oxidative stress by a combination of live blood analysis and urine testing. I use a test which measures MDA (malondialdeyhde), a byproduct of fat oxidation. The redder the sample, the more MDA is present and the more fat oxidation occurring.

- Candida diagnosis.

Some naturopaths will do a candida test which requires a drop or two of fingertip blood. The results take about ten minutes, and will determine the presence of anti-candida antibodies. This indicates that the organism *candida albicans* has overgrown and become pathogenic. Often this causes symptoms like thrush, but can cause milder vague symptoms as well such as digestive upset and skin rashes. Some people experience no symptoms. Overgrowth of candida indicates either a weakened immune system, or bowel dysbiosis.

- Urinary Indican test.

This is a test for bowel dysbiosis. It determines both the presence of abnormal bacteria in the gut, and also the degree of imbalance. Everyone I have tested for this in practice comes back positive to some degree. It is a condition of living in modern society. The test can turn negative though, once a detoxification and gut repair program has been followed.

The urine is mixed with reagents, and the colour changes. The deeper the colour, the higher the degree of dysbiosis. We test the urine for bowel dysbiosis because the kidneys eliminate a breakdown product of bacterial overgrowth, indoxyl sulfate. This substance absorbs into the bloodstream from the gut, and then passes through the kidneys and into the urine.

- Allergy tests and sensitivity tests.

Undetected allergies and sensitivities can cause excess inflammation in the body. We know that inflammation underlies many of the problems associates with PCOS, so minimising sources of inflammation, as well as supporting the body's natural anti-inflammatory processes is important.

It can be worthwhile to determine if you are allergic or reactive to anything. This can be done with certain types of blood tests and skin prick tests. There are immediate allergies and delayed allergies, so a negative result in one test does not rule out a different type of allergy, and does not rule out a 'sensitivity' or inflammatory reaction. A sensitivity is a reaction to a food or substance that doesn't involve production of antibodies by the immune system. Instead, a general inflammatory reaction is produced, along with various symptoms that may be difficult to attribute to the offending agent.

Supervised elimination diets can be useful, but require strict commitment for a number of weeks or months. Sometimes just eliminating some of the most common offenders (wheat, dairy, corn, soy, salicylates) for a couple of weeks and then reintroducing them one at a time can pinpoint common sensitivities. It is best to work with your health professional to determine what tests to have done.

Kinesiology is a non-invasive complementary therapy that can be worth trying, to investigate possible sensitivities. I find it to be quite accurate. It is based on 'muscle testing', where exposure to an offending substance causes a weakening of the muscles when tested. This is something best explained by watching and experiencing. Based on the muscular response to certain foods that you would normally eat, you can formulate a list of foods to avoid, and determine the accuracy of the results by documenting your symptoms (or reduction in symptoms) over time.

I have had a variety of tests done, and eliminating the offending foods or eating them less frequently has played a big role in my success. I encourage you to explore this option.

*   Not all naturopathic practitioners will perform the tests that have been mentioned, as many are not a standard part of naturopathic education. They are testing procedures that an individual practitioner may choose to learn if they wish. When finding a practitioner to perform some of these tests, make sure the person assessing your results is a qualified health professional as well, and not just a technician.

THE POWER OVER PCOS '7 STEP SOLUTION

Once you have assessed your state of health through a variety of means, you should have a good indication of what the priorities are and what your goals are. For example, if you are overweight or obese, you may choose to focus on a specific fat loss program first, as losing fat will greatly improve your symptoms and reduce the risks associated with PCOS.

As figure seven shows, you can choose to follow a fat loss program either on its own for a few months, or in conjunction with the 7 Step Solution for best results. Or you may simply like to see how you go with the 7 Step Solution first, as this will still cause changes in your body to make you more able to lose body fat, and for some people, this may be enough. For others, following a specific protocol for fat loss might be necessary to kick start things and increase the rate of fat loss.

The 7 Step Solution is suitable for both normal weight and overweight women, but since losing fat is a concern for many women with PCOS, I have added some extra information for boosting fat loss after the discussion of the 7 Step Solution.

The 7 Step Solution is based on seven key areas (see figure eight). I will list suggestions for you to implement for each key area, categorised as 'basic' or 'advanced'. I have arranged it this way in understanding that some of you reading this book will be newly diagnosed and haven't really started any treatment or dietary changes. Others may have been dealing with PCOS for years and feel you are already doing as many things as you can.

For those who are just starting, you may like to begin with only the 'basic' suggestions to prevent feeling overwhelmed. It is best for you to make small changes gradually, one step at a time.

For those who are already following a variety of guidelines, you may find that moving on to 'advanced' strategies will allow you to finally achieve success, or maybe there are some options in the basic category that you have not been following that you can start to implement.

The key word here is 'implementation'. It is no good reading about things, thinking "Oh, that's interesting, I must look into that one day". Your success depends not only on the acquiring of knowledge, but on the 'implementation' of this knowledge.

Figure 8: The categories of the 7 Step Solution

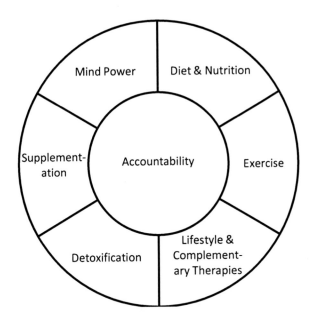

STEP ONE: DIET AND NUTRITION

BASIC SUGGESTIONS

- **Eat a low GI diet:**

GI stands for glycaemic index, which is a numbered ranking of foods based on how quickly that food raises your blood sugar. Low GI foods raise your blood sugar levels more slowly than high GI foods.

When you have PCOS, it is vital to eat foods with a low GI. Because sugar is absorbed into the bloodstream more slowly with low GI foods, less insulin needs to be produced. Lower insulin is desirable because too much insulin can stimulate the production of testosterone, the male hormone that is responsible for many of the symptoms of PCOS such as acne, excess hair, scalp hair loss, and menstrual irregularities. Insulin also has the effect of 'switching off' fat burning in cells, making it harder to lose weight.

Low GI eating can help to reduce your insulin levels and balance hormones, keep your energy levels stable for longer, and reduce sweet cravings. Try eating lower GI alternatives such as apples, pears, oats, basmati rice, sweet potato, and lentils. Avoid or reduce white and wholemeal breads, potato, jasmine rice, and added sugar. When baking, use xylitol instead of sugar. Xylitol has a GI of only 7. If you haven't already, I recommend investing in a book that lists the GI values of a large variety of foods. Don't assume what the GI of a food is, look it up! You can find out more about the GI and various books that are available by visiting www.glycemicindex.com.

You can also go a step further by eating a low **GL** diet. This stands for glycaemic load. This is a combination of the GI of a food and the amount of carbohydrates it contains. So by eating a food that is low GI *and* low GL, you are not only slowing the *rate* of glucose absorption into the bloodstream, you are also reducing the *amount* of glucose entering the bloodstream over the course of the day. This reduces your demand for insulin, which can lower excess hormones and help you to burn body fat more effectively.

- **Balance your food intake:**

You may have been told to "eat a balanced diet", but what exactly does this mean? It basically means having a wide variety of foods and varying the types of proteins you eat, and eating plenty of vegetables and fruits. Your diet should be based largely around vegetables and plant foods, and you should be eating sources of 'complete protein' every day.

Complete protein supplies all the essential amino acids that build new cells and proteins in the body. Usual sources are animal products such as eggs, lean meats, chicken, and fish. Vegetarian sources include soy, and the combining of foods such as grains and vegetables with legumes. Nuts are a good source of protein, and if you combine almonds, brazils, and cashews, this makes a complete protein. Just remember ABC! (Almonds, Brazils, Cashews).

The type of fat you eat is important. Although fat is energy dense (high in calories), fats are essential for health. Saturated fats are to be reduced, such as those from meat, full fat dairy products, chicken skin, and butter. Trans fats are also to be reduced, or better yet, avoided. Trans fats are mostly in foods such as biscuits or cookies, crackers and crispbreads, processed cakes, slices, pastries, and margarines. When buying meats, get lean cuts and trim off all visible fat. Peel skin off chicken before cooking. Avoid fatty sausages.

The fats to focus on are those that are high in the essential omega 3 and omega 6 fats. Fats to enjoy are found in foods such as avocado, nuts, seeds such as pumpkin seeds and linseeds/flaxseeds, olive oil, rice bran oil, sunflower oil, and fish. Use avocado as a sandwich spread instead of butter or margarine, sprinkle chopped walnuts on a salad, cook with olive or rice bran oil, and eat fish three times a week.

A balanced diet also contains enough fibre. Fibre is what provides roughage or bulk in the digestive tract, helping to clear the bowel of waste and stimulating the contractions in the gut wall. It also keeps you feeling full.

Soluble fibre absorbs water and often slows the absorption of glucose, as well as helping to reduce cholesterol re-absorption. Soluble fibre is in foods such as oats and apples. Psyllium husks are also a good source. Try a couple of teaspoons a day to keep bowels regular. Whenever you increase your fibre intake you must also increase your water intake, otherwise the fibre will not work and you will feel blocked up.

Water is another component of a balanced diet. It is the only liquid you need to drink. If you don't like the 'taste' of it, just treat it like a medicine and gulp it down! You will get used to it and after a while probably crave it. The body loses an average of two litres a day (equivalent to about 8 glasses). Your body can make a small amount each day, and you also get some from food, but the best way to stay hydrated is to drink water. There's no escaping this one... just do it!

Try to break up your food intake to three main meals, and two snacks in between. Don't eat within two hours of sleeping or your sleep will suffer and you will be more likely to store fat. If you tend to leave cooking till the last minute, and you reach for convenience food instead, spend some time on the weekend making up a few meals to freeze for during the week. Vegetable soup is good, as are lean salmon and vegetable patties. Freeze some cooked chicken strips and then add to a bowl of salad greens and a small amount of low GI rice with a lemon, chilli, and olive oil dressing. Start experimenting and you will be surprised at the quick and easy meals you can come up with that are healthy. If you lack motivation, get a healthy cookbook and follow the instructions. Plan ahead too, so you know what ingredients you need and how much time you will need to prepare.

- **Go natural:**

Modern food is heavily processed and missing vital nutrients. I am surprised that some foods are even considered food when you read the label. They seem to consist of mostly numbers that indicate additives such as flavour enhancers, preservatives, colours, flavours, with a bit of added starch for substance!

Base your diet around simple, basic, natural food. Good quality food, as fresh as possible. Grow some of your own vegetables if you can, and shop from small local markets. Snack on fruits and nuts, make your own healthy low GI muffins for treats, use bread without preservatives, drink only water or natural juices or herbal teas, eat free range organic eggs, and make your own healthy sauces and dressings. Limit processed foods from packets and fast food outlets. Get used to reading labels, go for foods without added flavour enhancers, preservatives, colours, and flavours. You will be providing your body with more nutrients by eating naturally, and you will reduce your toxic load. It is all about getting back to basics. Your body will thank you for it! Learn more about additive free eating at www.fedupwithfoodadditives.info.

ADVANCED SUGGESTIONS

- **Go organic:**

Whenever possible, purchase organic produce to reduce your toxic load. This is especially important for meat and poultry, which may have remnants of antibiotics or hormone disrupting chemicals. If your fruit and vegetables are not organic, make sure you wash them well, and don't eat the skin as this will have had the highest exposure to chemical pesticides. Take advantage of the many organic home delivery services available. Organic food tends to taste better, and is better for you.

- **Reduce or avoid dairy, or use only A2 dairy products:**

Many people have improved their health by avoiding dairy products. If you have grown up with milk on cereal, cheese on crackers, ice cream, and frothy cappuccinos, you may find this suggestion hard to implement. I was the same, I was in a sense 'addicted' to dairy (and you will find out soon that this is in fact true). I absolutely loved cheese and would eat it daily, I had milk every day, and as a child I have memories of being treated to ice creams and milkshakes when out. When it was suggested to me that my health and symptoms may improve by avoiding dairy, I freaked out! "There's no way I can give that up" I thought.

Well, now it is a different story. I don't feel a 'need' for dairy products anymore. Once I started reducing them and eventually avoiding them, my health improved. The hay fever and allergic rhinitis symptoms I thought were due to my cat disappeared. My digestion improved, and my mood improved. I was also able to lose fat more easily.

Problems with dairy are due to a few things. Firstly, the majority of people as they get older develop some degree of lactose intolerance. This is because the enzyme that digests lactose naturally reduces with age. I'm not talking about old age, this natural reduction starts to occur in infancy. Breast milk contains some lactose, but once a baby is weaned the enzyme lactase starts to decline. Most children are then put onto cow's milk, but consider this... we humans are the only mammals to drink another mammals milk! This is just my opinion, but somehow it doesn't seem natural.

We have been brought up to think that if we don't have our three serves of dairy each day, we won't get enough calcium and are therefore at risk of osteoporosis. But there are countries that don't have dairy and don't have a high incidence of osteoporosis. Yes, dairy is high in calcium and other nutrients, but calcium is not the only preventative factor in osteoporosis.

Dairy milk is a natural 'growth promoter'. Its purpose is to help the baby cow grow. In humans, there are some concerns that it may stimulate the production of insulin-like growth factors[11], that encourage growth and fat storage. We also know that raised levels of insulin like growth factor-1 seem to be responsible for many of the consequences of PCOS in addition to raised insulin[12].

Despite the low glycaemic index of many dairy products, some research indicates that dairy products may result in an increase in insulin levels, which is bad news for PCOS. You can read some of the research on this webpage:
http://www.ajcn.org/cgi/content/full/74/1/96

Apart from these factors, the main problem with dairy seems to be in regards to one of its proteins called **casein**. More specifically; *A1 beta-casein*. This form of casein is contained in dairy products in most of the western world. Other parts of the world such as Africa, Asia, and some parts of southern Europe, have dairy products that contain a different form of casein – A2 beta casein, which does not seem to be linked to health problems.

Thousands of years ago all dairy was A2, but due to a genetic mutation, some cows started producing A1 beta casein. The difference between the two is just one amino acid (amino acids are the building blocks of proteins). This difference is quite significant, as it means that when A1 beta casein is digested, it releases what's called a 'peptide' (small protein). This peptide is very resistant to further breakdown and usually gets absorbed into the bloodstream intact, especially in people with leaky gut syndrome or increased intestinal permeability. The name of this peptide is **beta-casomorphin-7 (BCM7)**. It has opioid (narcotic properties) in the brain[13] (similar to morphine), which may explain why some people can become 'addicted' to eating foods such as dairy. Gluten, the protein found in wheat, rye, barely, and sometimes oats, also releases an opioid similar to BCM7. Eliminating these foods has shown great benefits for many children with autism, including my own son.

Epidemiological studies show that societies in which A1 dairy is a major part of the diet, have a higher incidence of diseases such as heart disease, type 1 diabetes, autoimmune diseases, autism, and schizophrenia. Considering PCOS may be linked with an increased risk of heart disease, it is wise to investigate this possible link between dairy and heart disease.

Before jumping to conclusions about the dairy issue, or agreeing with the dairy industry that there is no strong evidence, I recommend you do your own reading on the matter. The book 'Devil in the milk' by Keith Woodford *(2007. Craig Potton Publishing New Zealand),* is an excellent publication that discusses both sides of the story in an evidence based way. It is compelling reading, and has convinced me that we should be switching from A1 to A2 milk, or avoiding dairy protein completely. The book goes into detail about the health effects of BCM7, some proven, some still undergoing research. Some of them include:

- In vitro (test tube), BCM7 has strong oxidant properties. Remember, oxidative stress is a situation in which there is too much 'oxidation'. If BCM7 is an oxidant, dairy would add to this oxidative stress. It can oxidise low density lipoprotein (LDL), also known as the 'bad cholesterol'. This is how heart disease can start, oxidised fat is deposited into artery walls.

- BCM7 can slow the rate of waste passage through the digestive tract, and may contribute to constipation in some people. However, this can be counteracted in some people by the effect of lactose intolerance causing diarrhea.

- French and Spanish researchers have shown in vitro that BCM7 increases mucous secretions by over 69% compared to controls. This may explain why some people report more symptoms of congestion when they eat dairy.

- BCM7 can compromise immune function. It also has a very similar structure to the GLUT2 molecule in the pancreas. This molecule transports glucose into the cells in the pancreas that produce insulin. The immune system can create antibodies that attack BCM7, but because it is similar to GLUT2, the immune system can get confused and also attack GLUT2, possibly damaging the insulin-producing cells in the pancreas.

Dairy is a controversial issue, but an important one to investigate. It is not in the scope of this book to go into much more detail, but I suggest you consider looking into this issue as a possible way for you to improve your health further and prevent future risks of PCOS.

- **Determine foods that cause allergic or inflammatory reactions and avoid them:**

Many people go about their day, unaware that they have a food allergy or intolerance. Undiagnosed food intolerances can be responsible for a large variety of symptoms. Reactions may occur instantly or after a few days, so the culprit can be hard to pin point unless a strict elimination diet is done or certain tests are performed.

If you are not feeling like you are getting the best results possible from your diet and treatments, I recommend investigating possible reactions to foods. These reactions may include a definite immune response where antibodies are produced, or a more general inflammatory reaction.

You could start by having one or two allergy tests for both immediate and delayed reactions. Speak to your doctor about getting a skin prick test done, or a blood test to determine antibodies to common foods.

Some health practitioners also perform an allergy test for delayed reactions involving the IgG antibody. This test uses only a few drops of blood from the fingertip, and tests your reactions to about one hundred different foods.

There are also various other testing procedures that some health practitioners can provide, to determine *sensitivities* to foods, as opposed to *allergies*. One such test is the Meridian Stress Assessment System (MSAS) – www.biomeridian.com

Kinesiology is another technique, that when performed by an experienced practitioner, may be able to pick up reactions to various foods and substances. It is useful as it does not involve the taking of blood.

- **Reduce/avoid wheat:**

Wheat is a common problem for many people because of the fact that it is very processed these days, and is naturally a hard to digest grain. It is high in gluten, a protein that some people react to (e.g.: those with coeliac disease), and produces a molecule with narcotic properties in the brain.

I have discovered through my research that many women with PCOS also suffer from digestive complaints. If you experience stomach bloating, I suggest trying a wheat free diet for a week or so to see if it improves. In clinical practice I find this is the most common symptom of wheat intolerance. Wheat can also cause other symptoms in certain people, such as reflux, wheezing, skin rashes, and mood changes.

For some people, it is not just wheat, but all gluten containing grains that cause problems. If you are having digestive symptoms and have ruled out coeliac disease, first try going wheat free for a week or so, then if there is no change, go gluten free (no rye, barley, oats). The other way of doing it is to try avoiding all gluten for three weeks, then reintroducing one grain at a time, starting with oats. Then if there is no reaction, reintroduce barley, then rye, then wheat.

- **Eat a Paleolithic diet:**

If you have a particularly severe case of PCOS, especially if you suffer with acne, you may have success with a Paleolithic diet. This can be difficult to follow in modern society, but can be a very effective and healthy way of eating. It involves eating a diet along the lines of what our ancestors, the hunter-gatherers ate.

It is based on simple, fresh foods including lean meats, poultry, fish, eggs, vegetables (except potatoes), fruits, and good oils. It avoids dairy, cereal grains, legumes, soy, and any processed foods. If you feel you have exhausted all avenues and are not 100% happy with your results, I recommend a trial period of this diet for a minimum of thirty days. You will need to plan and prepare before starting, as when you begin you will most likely experience some withdrawal effects and cravings for carbohydrates. I recommend reading Dr Loren Cordain's book 'The Paleo Diet', or 'The Dietary Cure For Acne' which will give you all the information you need to follow this way of eating. Information can be found at:

www.thepaleodiet.com
www.dietaryacnecure.com

Remember though, that there may be certain foods permitted on this diet (such as certain vegetables), that you may have an unknown intolerance to. Finding out your individual intolerances through testing procedures is a good idea first, to make sure you get the best results.

STEP TWO: EXERCISE

BASIC SUGGESTIONS

- **Increase incidental exercise:**

The more your body is active, the more fat you will burn, and the healthier your whole body will be. Even if you are of a normal weight, exercise is still very important. It strengthens your heart and lungs, tones your muscles, makes you more sensitive to insulin, improves your mood, increases energy, and increases circulation. If there was a pill for that everyone would be taking it! Exercise is one of the simplest and effective strategies for a healthier body.

Have a look at your lifestyle and work out where the opportunities lie for being more active. Any chance you get to move around, take it. Walk to work if nearby, get off one stop earlier from the train or bus, take ten minutes on your lunch break to go for a walk, take the stairs instead of the lift, when watching television, get up on the commercial breaks and move around the house or do some push-ups and sit-ups. You get the picture? Any movement is better than none. Don't wait for 'time' to exercise, make it part of your day.

- **Use a pedometer:**

A pedometer or a step counter is a very motivating tool to help you get enough activity each day. It attaches to the waist of your pants, skirt, or belt, and registers each step you take by the movement of your legs. Experts say to aim for around 10,000 steps each day, or more if you are trying to lose weight.

Give it a go one day with your normal routine, and see how many steps you clock up. If you are under 10,000, then make a plan on how to increase your steps. Don't worry if you don't get to 10,000 steps every single day, as long as you are clocking up at least 70,000 steps over the course of a week, which is the main thing. Some days are always more active than others. Pedometers are very useful tools to assess your activity levels, but to also motivate you to exercise more. (Just remember to remove it each time you go to the bathroom, I have heard many cases of pedometers 'accidentally' falling into the toilet!).

- **Do 'interval exercise' three times a week:**

Interval exercise helps you to build stronger muscles, a more efficient heart, and a greater lung capacity, which helps you burn excess calories and fat. Studies show it may be more effective than standard aerobic exercise.

In the past, society has been advised to perform aerobic exercise in order to lose weight and keep healthy. Aerobic exercise involves moving around at a moderate to high intensity for a duration of between thirty and sixty minutes on average. Now, it is known to be better to break up your exercise with alternating periods of low intensity and moderate to high intensity exertion periods. This is known as interval exercise. Just ten to twenty minutes of interval exercise, a few times a week, often gives greater benefits than long duration aerobic exercise.

An example of an interval routine:

Type of exercise: walking on a treadmill
Duration: fifteen minutes
Routine:
- Walk slowly for one minute to warm up.
- Walk slightly faster for two minutes.
- Walk slowly for two minutes.
- Walk faster for two minutes.
- Walk slowly for two minutes.
- Walk faster for two minutes.
- Walk slowly for one minute.
- Walk faster for one minute.
- Walk slowly for two minutes.

As you get fitter you can increase the intensity of the exertion periods, and shorten the intervals (eg: sixty seconds, forty five seconds)

Plan ahead and mark in your diary the best times for you to exercise. If you make an 'appointment' with yourself you will be more likely to stick to it. Also, do exercise that you enjoy, here are some options to try:

- ☐ Walking outdoors or on a treadmill

- ☐ Low intensity walking, with bursts of jogging/running for 30-60 seconds at a time, every 5 minutes

- ☐ Light jogging, varying your speed and incline

- ☐ Exercise classes

- ☐ Exercise DVD's

- ☐ Dancing classes – jazz, contemporary, salsa, hip hop, African

- ☐ Hiking

- ☐ Cycling, outdoors or on an exercise bike

- ☐ Swimming

- ☐ Rowing, outdoors or on a rowing machine

- ☐ Hire a personal trainer

ADVANCED SUGGESTIONS

- **Do a combination of interval, resistance, and flexibility exercises:**

Exercise that moves your body around like walking is important, but for PCOS, resistance exercise is just as important if you want to improve your insulin sensitivity, body composition, and balance your hormones. Resistance exercise strengthens and builds your muscles. Muscles burn fat about fifty percent of the time, so by having more muscle tissue, you have an increased ability to burn body fat, even while you sleep.

Resistance exercise includes anything that puts a stress on your muscles. Anything that makes them contract and provide force against a resistance or weight. Each day you are doing resistance exercise without realising, for example, the act of holding your head up straight all day. You do it without thinking, because you learned to do it as a baby, and now it is easy. It is the same with other muscles, if you use them regularly, it will become easier and easier to use them. Strong muscles not only help you burn fat, and give you a toned and sculpted appearance, but they also support your joints and bones, making you less likely to suffer from falls and accidents as you get older.

When you do resistance exercise (which contracts the muscles), you need to balance it out with flexibility exercises (which stretch the muscles). This helps to prevent injuries and cramps, and makes it easier for your body to move around each day.

This is what I suggest as a general guide for exercise:

- **Interval exercise:** 15 to 20 minutes, at least 3 to 4 times per week.

- **Resistance exercise:** Every third day, or work on one major muscle group every day, leaving at least 2 days between working on a particular muscle group. This is because muscle actually grows and become stronger with rest.

- Examples:

    - Do a whole body resistance workout at home or at the gym every third day.

- OR

    - Work on one major muscle group each day. Day1: upper body, Day 2: abdominals and core strength, Day 3: lower body. Day 4: rest day, or start with upper body again.

Flexibility exercise: Stretch the muscles gently and slowly after each resistance workout, or do a complete body flexibility session several times per week (e.g.: yoga, stretching).

If you get bored easily, rotate the types of exercise you do. Exercise outdoors if possible, and use the services of a trainer if you need extra support and motivation.

STEP THREE: LIFESTYLE AND COMPLEMENTARY THERAPIES

BASIC SUGGESTIONS

- **Create your ideal healthy lifestyle:**

Have a think about whether you are truly happy with the way your life is from day to day. Are you focused too much on work or study, or are you bored and in need of more excitement and fun? Take a step back and look at this issue. Look at what you have done and achieved in this past week. At the end of your life will you be happy with how things turned out? Or are there things in your life that you have been putting off, or maybe you feel trapped in your current situation. If you are not satisfied, work out what it is you truly want and make a plan to create the lifestyle that YOU want to live. Create a balance between work, study, and leisure. Take time for yourself, and time to spend with others.

Life does not *happen* to you, you *create* it. So take steps to consciously create the life you want. You will be happier and healthier for it.

- **Get adequate sleep:**

Sleep quantity and quality is an often overlooked factor in the state of your health. If we spend one third of our lives asleep then it must be pretty important! Sleep research is bringing us some exciting discoveries related to health, and I feel it is a crucial part of any plan to improve one's health.

A lack of sleep causes many negative effects, more than just feeling tired and cranky. It actually reduces your ability to balance your blood sugar and insulin levels, and over time can make you more prone to diabetes[14]. Lack of sleep can make you feel hungrier and make you more likely to put on weight. This is partly because it reduces levels of the hormone 'leptin'[15]. Leptin normally makes you feel satisfied and full, so when it is reduced, you are more likely to feel hunger.

Sleep research has told us that people who get an average of eight hours of quality sleep each night, tend to live longer than those who get more or less. So don't think you have to burn the midnight oil to get *more* done, because it may mean you actually get *less* done if you don't live as long!

Women with PCOS are at an increased risk of sleep apnoea, a condition in which you stop breathing for short periods of time, repeatedly throughout the night. These short periods of time add up, and result in many hours of lost sleep each week. Sleep apnoea has many possible consequences including weight gain, diabetes, high blood pressure, heart attack, stroke, and car accidents from falling asleep at the wheel. If you are always feeling tired throughout the day, un-refreshed after sleep, or have high blood pressure that is hard to control, it is **vital** that you get checked for sleep apnoea. It could save your (or someone else's) life. Diagnosis usually involves spending the night in a sleep clinic, attached to electrodes. It may be uncomfortable but it is only one night of your life.

If you have trouble getting to sleep, or you want to optimise your sleep, try these tips:

- Have a regular routine each evening and go to bed at the same time.
- The earlier you get to sleep, the better your sleep quality will be. Aim to be asleep by no later than 10:30pm.

- Turn the lights off and use candle light for two hours before sleep. It will allow your body to produce melatonin, the sleep hormone.
- When you get up in the morning, expose yourself to bright white light, like sunshine. There are even light boxes you can get for those who live in countries where there is not much sunshine. Light will set your body clock and the earlier you get it, the earlier you will be able to fall asleep.
- Don't exercise within two hours of sleep, it will stimulate your body and mind. An exception is yoga or stretching, this can often help you to get a good sleep.
- Avoid caffeine and alcohol within five hours of sleep. Better yet, avoid these substances completely!
- Take a magnesium supplement. If you wake often throughout the night, you may have a magnesium deficiency. Take 150mg* with your evening meal, and another 150mg an hour before bed and see if this helps.
- *150mg of *elemental* magnesium. The label may say something like magnesium citrate 500mg, but this is not the amount of magnesium, this is the magnesium *and* the citrate together. Usually in brackets it will say something like (total magnesium 100mg).
- Listen to a guided relaxation CD before bed.
- If you still have trouble, visit a natural health professional for advice. Herbs like *zizyphus* and *passionflower* can help.

If you have a baby or young children, it can obviously be hard to get a good night's sleep if they wake throughout the night. This can be very exhausting (trust me, I know, my son didn't sleep through the night until age five!).

Adopt a good routine for them, dim the lights in the hour or two before their bedtime, and avoid stimulating story books before bed. If your child is getting older and still waking throughout the night, there are professionals out there that specialise in this. Take any help that is available, and make sure you have time during the day to rest. For persistent night wakers, I would also investigate possible food allergies or intolerances. Dairy can be a culprit for many children.

- **Avoid destructive lifestyle habits:**

If you are a smoker, you MUST take action to remove this destructive habit from your life. Cigarettes are highly toxic. I won't go into detail as I know that you know they are not healthy. I also know they are highly addictive and that beating any addiction is no easy feat. There is help out there, take it. Get support and make a plan to quit. Some people have found the book "The easy way to stop smoking" by Allen Carr helpful.

Alcohol is another factor that can affect your health. Although the current recommendations suggest alcohol in moderation, if you are dealing with any health condition I suggest avoiding it completely. It will only add to your body's load. Alcohol is used as an energy source and will prevent glucose or sugar being used up until the alcohol has been metabolised. It can therefore affect your blood sugar balance, and can also lead to weight gain. It takes your liver away from other important tasks, it depletes good bacteria in the gut, and can even increase your testosterone levels, something you don't want in PCOS!

Another addiction that often goes unnoticed is emotional eating. This is very common in PCOS. Food is sometimes seen as a way of making us feel good, or replacing something that is missing from our lives. If this addiction is not dealt with, no amount of good dietary advice will help. The causes and triggers of your emotional eating habit must be discovered and addressed to truly improve.

Before you reach for food as an emotional reaction, be aware that you are about to do this and think "Am I really hungry?", "Is this food really going to nourish my body?". Have a glass of water and wait half an hour and see how you feel. If emotional eating is a problem for you, I recommend visiting www.healyourhunger.com .

ADVANCED SUGGESTIONS

- **Incorporate complementary therapies into your life:**

There are many natural therapies available that are a beneficial adjunct to your lifestyle and health plan. If you were to choose one, I would suggest a chiropractic or osteopathic assessment and treatment if required. This will assess whether any of the bones in your spine are out of alignment. This can occur with daily life, from movement, poor posture, sleeping position, stress, exercise, weak muscles, and injury. Many people have spines that are not in proper alignment and are unaware of this. Other bones can be misaligned too, such as the ribs, collarbone, shoulder blades, and pelvis.

The result of the misalignment is that pressure is placed on certain nerves coming from the spinal cord, stimulating or inhibiting them. This can result in malfunction in the organ supplied by the particular nerve. For example, if nerves near your lower spine are affected, your reproductive organs may malfunction.

It is extremely worthwhile getting a full assessment done by a qualified practitioner. Good structure is the framework of the body, and we need to support it.

Other complementary therapies you may find beneficial are:

- **Acupuncture:**

Fine needles are placed in the skin at certain 'meridian points' to balance the flow of energy or chi in the body. Acupuncture has gained increasing acceptance and popularity in society, and it is known for its benefits with pain control. It may also help to balance hormones, reduce stress perception, and improve the functioning of the whole body.

For women's health, acupuncture has shown particular benefits for increasing fertility, regulating cycles, and reducing morning sickness. A number of treatments may be required. Make sure you see a qualified practitioner who uses disposable needles.

- **Massage:**

Most people find massage enjoyable. It can form a valuable part of your health treatment plan by reducing stress, improving mood, easing sore muscles, providing 'time out', stimulating circulation and waste elimination, and certain massage techniques can even help to break down cellulite. Most of all, it just feels good! If you have never had a massage, or haven't had one in a long time, why not make a booking? You deserve it!

- **Reflexology:**

Reflexology stimulates certain points on the soles of the feet, and sometimes the hands and ears. These points are said to correlate to certain parts of the body. Tender spots may be felt in areas that relate to a part of the body that is out of balance, stimulation of these areas may help to balance out these parts of the body.

- **Reiki & energetic healing:**

Reiki is an energetic therapy that aims to restore vibrational balance in the energy systems of the body. The practitioner may or may not have physical contact with you. They are trained to be attuned to the sensation of energy in another person's body, and to be able to use their own energy to balance that of the patient. There are also various other forms of energetic healing techniques available.

Remember, energy is something that can affect which genes in a cell's DNA are activated. A positive energy will nurture the body, negative energies are destructive.

- **Hypnosis:**

Hypnosis with a qualified practitioner, or with a self hypnosis CD, can be very useful for dealing with specific issues such as fear, low self esteem, emotional eating, anxiety...etc. If there is a specific thing bothering you that you feel you have no control over, hypnosis may be able to 're-program' your subconscious mind so that you can regain control.

STEP FOUR: DETOXIFICATION

BASIC SUGGESTIONS

- **Reduce exposure to toxins:**

You can't totally eliminate toxins from your environment, but you can greatly reduce your load. You may be surprised at the changes you feel after reducing your exposure. Here are some ways to reduce your toxic load. The more of them you decide to implement, the better:

Personal:

- Use natural shampoo and conditioner, avoid those with sodium laureth sulfate.

- Use natural skin care, free of chemical preservatives like parabens.

- Try mineral make-up as an alternative to make-up with chemical ingredients.

- Use natural shower gels and liquid soaps, without sodium laureth sulfate and formaldehyde.

- Use natural body lotion, moisturizers, and sunscreens.

- Use sanitary products made with natural fibres.

- Use natural plant based toothpaste.

Household:

- Avoid synthetic cleaning sprays, dishwashing powders, dishwashing liquids, and laundry products. They are not necessary. Use natural alternatives or home made cleaning solutions including bicarbonate of soda and lemon juice. The Australian products; tea tree oil and eucalyptus oil also make good cleaners when diluted, especially when added to washing machines. There are various books available that show you how to easily and cheaply clean your home without chemicals. Try 'Chemical Free Home' by Robyn Stewart.

- Allow your home to get fresh air as much as possible. If you live in a polluted city, you might like to invest in an air cleaner, to remove airborne chemicals and germs.

- Use indoor plants, especially in areas where there is radiation from computers and other electronic equipment.

- Use carpets and rugs with natural fibres, or go for natural wood floorboards.

- If possible, when parking your car in a garage that is attached to your house, don't close the garage door right away. Leave it open for as long as possible so as to not enclose the toxins that will still be seeping out from the exhaust.

- Follow the dietary advice in this book, eat natural based foods and wash fruit and vegetables before eating. Many chemicals you are exposed to are actually consumed.

- Purchase a stainless steel water bottle instead of using a plastic one. If you do use plastic bottles, rinse well before use, and refill the water if it is left too long in the bottle.

- Store food in glass or stainless steel containers (but don't put glass in the freezer, it will explode!). Don't reheat food in plastic containers, if you do reheat food, use ceramic or glass containers.

- Reduce the use of your microwave oven. Or, consider getting rid of it. Plan meals ahead of time so you can defrost meat or chicken in the refrigerator overnight instead of the microwave, and reheat meals on a stove.

- Consider minimising the use of non-stick cookware. Use stainless steel cookware, and olive oil or rice bran oil to prevent sticking.

*See www.resources.poweroverpcos.com to find out

recommended sources of natural products.

- **Take supplements to enhance detoxification:**

Supplements will be discussed in step five. A good nutritional supplement program will provide your body with an optimal amount of nutrients required for overall health and detoxification. There are also more specific supplements and herbal options that can enhance your detoxification ability.

ADVANCED SUGGESTIONS

- **Do a proper detoxification program, and repeat it every six to twelve months:**

There are various 'detox kits' available in health food shops, but most are not a long term solution, and many are put together in a way that is not logical or based on how the body actually works. I recommend doing a safe detox program with a qualified and experienced practitioner who uses tried and tested protocols. You can also follow this general detox program that I have layed out for you.

*Cautions:

- Do not start a detox program if you are pregnant or breastfeeding, are currently sick, have recently had surgery, or are on blood thinning medications, without professional guidance and supervision.

- If you are trying to conceive, you may start a detox program, but you will need to stop taking the detox supplements if you find out you are pregnant. It is usually best to avoid getting pregnant while doing the detox program, and it can actually be quite an effective pre-conception program to prepare your body for conceiving.

- If you are on a lot of different medications, please follow the guidance of your healthcare professional before starting a detox program.

- The detox program I use usually lasts for a minimum of seven weeks, but sometimes up to twelve weeks, depending on the individual.

A proper detox program will consist of three stages, generally described as:

1. **Weed**
2. **Seed & Feed**
3. **Speed**

1. The **weed** stage involves getting rid of the overgrowth of bad bacteria and other microorganisms, as well as built up waste matter from the digestive tract.

2. The **seed** and **feed** stage involves replenishing the good bacteria (seeding), and healing the lining if the digestive tract (feeding). Feeding also involves creating an optimal environment for the growth of the good bacteria.

3. The **speed** stage simply means speeding up waste and toxin elimination through the liver.

These stages are supported by the use of specific supplements. See the resources page at www.resources.poweroverpcos.com to find out my recommended sources of the detox supplements.

While taking the supplements as part of the detox program, it is vital that you also reduce your toxic load as outlined previously, and follow the basic dietary suggestions in Step One, with the addition of:

- Avoiding caffeine, coffee, tea

- Avoiding alcohol

- Avoiding dairy, or only eating plain yoghurt, goat's milk, goat's fetta, and mozzarella cheese, which are less reactive.
- Avoiding potato

- Avoiding more than ¼ cup of dried fruit daily

- Avoiding processed meats like bacon and ham

- Avoiding battered or crumbed fish and chicken

- Avoiding tuna

- Avoiding baked beans, peanuts, and peanut butter

- Avoiding added sugar

- Avoiding wheat and rye

Supplement regime for detox program:

*Stage One: usually 3 to 4 weeks

<u>1. Initial colon cleanse:</u> first 6 days

Take an oxygen based colon cleanser as directed, for at least six days. This will liquefy any built up or compacted waste matter in the digestive tract that has accumulated over the years. You should aim for three to five bowel movements each day while on this product. You will be able to carry out your normal activities, but you might like to start the cleanse on a weekend or when you have a day or two free, so you can see how your body responds to it. It will not give you diarrhoea as such, but will simply melt away any dried waste matter that is stuck in the bowel.

<u>2. Anti-microbial herbal formula</u>: minimum of 2 weeks, after the initial colon cleanse.

Use a herbal formula designed to have broad anti-microbial properties. A naturopath or herbalist can help you with this, or find a good quality formula that contains:

- Wormwood (Artemisia annua). Minimum of 2000mg daily.
- Black walnut (Juglans nigra). At least 3000mg daily.
- Olive leaf (Olea europaea). 1000mg to 3000mg daily.
- Oregano oil (Origanum vulgare).
- Ginger (Zingiber officinale)

In addition, there are other ingredients that can be good adjuncts to the above herbs:

- Barberry (Berberis vulgaris)
- Gentian (Gentiana lutea)
- Cinnamon (Cinnamomum zeylanicum)
- Thyme oil (Thymus vulgaris)
- Aniseed (Pimpinella anisum)
- Oregon grape (Berberis aquifolium)

Take the herbs as directed, usually twice per day (eg: breakfast and lunch is best). The dosage will depend on how much of each herb is contained in the formula. Several tablets may be needed to achieve the therapeutic doses suggested for the main herbs.

The following supplements are optional for stage one:

3. Prebiotic formula: minimum of 2 weeks, to support growth of good bacteria and encourage a healthy environment in the digestive tract.

Prebiotics provide food for good bacteria to survive. This can help reduce any wind or digestive upset that may occasionally occur when taking an anti-microbial formula. Examples of prebiotic ingredients are inulin, acacia, Jerusalem artichoke (helianthus tuberosis), and two sources of glyconutrients called arabinogalactans and galacto-oligosaccharides.

Don't confuse them with <u>pro</u>biotics, probiotics are the good bacteria themselves, prebiotics are the food for the good bacteria.

4. <u>Saccharomyces boulardii (cerevisiae):</u> minimum of 2 weeks to reduce candida overgrowth and manage dysbiosis.

Also known as SB, saccharomyces boulardii is actually a beneficial yeast that has anti-microbial functions, can prevent traveller's diarrheoa, and can eliminate excess candida overgrowth. Candida albicans overgrowth is a common occurrence, and if symptomatic it can result in thrush, skin rashes, a 'fuzzy' feeling in the head, or digestive complaints. A therapeutic dose can be taken in stage one of the detox, and sometimes stage two as well, as it can help create an optimal environment for good bacteria to grow.

If you are prone to thrush or digestive upsets, SB is a must for your detox program.

*Stage Two: usually 2 weeks

<u>1. Gut repair formula:</u>

Usually a powder that is mixed with a drink or combined with a low GI cereal, a good gut repair formula will have the following ingredients:

- Glutamine.
- Aloe vera juice powder (from the inner leaf juice)
Those two ingredients can also work synergistically with:

- Slippery elm powder
- Licorice root (deglycyrrhizinised)
- n-acetyl-d-glucosamine

Glutamine will provide a source of energy for the cells lining the gut, aloe vera has anti-inflammatory and healing effects on the gut tissue, slippery elm has fantastic soothing and healing effects, licorice root is anti-inflammatory and healing to the mucous membrane of the gut, and glucosamine has a tissue regenerating and anti-inflammatory effect.

2. Probiotic formula:

Once you have weeded out the bad bugs, you need to replenish the good bugs! High doses of different probiotics should be taken at this stage, and you may choose to maintain digestive health after the detox, by taking a probiotic formula every day at a maintenance dose, to keep dysbiosis at bay.

You need to get a good quality probiotic that is acid resistant so it won't break down in the stomach. You also need a quality strain of a probiotic species that will actually 'colonise' the gut and not just pass through. Eating yoghurt is not enough to replace good bacteria, and drinking special probiotic drinks you can find at the supermarket is not enough either. Probiotic supplements that guarantee a certain amount of bacteria per capsule are the way to go. Make sure your probiotic has both the lactobacillus and bifidobacterium species. There are several different types of each species, the main ones to look for are lactobacillus acidophilus, and bifidobacterium lactis or bifidus.

For stage two of the detox I would suggest taking a minimum of two capsules per day, depending on the individual formula, and depending on the individual. Also, you must keep probiotics in the refrigerator to maintain their viability.
The following supplements are optional for stage two:

3. Saccharomyces boulardii (cerevisiae):

You may continue SB for a couple more weeks if you were taking it in stage one, or if you weren't, you may choose to take it now to maximise the benefits of your program.

4. Lactobacillus plantarum:

This is a specific type of probiotic that reduces inflammation. You may choose to take this in addition to a general probiotic formula, especially if you have suffered with digestive complaints, food intolerances, or have a severe case of PCOS, which is associated with inflammation. This can often prevent inflammatory reactions in the gut before they take hold.

*Stage Three: usually 2 – 4 weeks

1. Herbs and Vegetables for detoxification:

There are some great tablet formulas that support liver detoxification. Make sure your formula has:

- St. Mary's Thistle (silybum marianum), also known as milk thistle. Minimum of 5000mg daily.

Other synergistic herbs and vegetables that enhance liver detoxification include:

- Globe artichoke (cynara scolymus)
- Schizandra (schizandra chinensis)
- Bupleurum (bupleurum falcatum)
- Broccoli (brassica oleracea)
- Green tea (camellia sinensis)
- Grape seed (vitis vinifera)

- Turmeric (curcuma longa)
- Beetroot (beta vulgaris)
- Pomegranate (punica granatum)
- Dandelion (taraxacum officinale)

2. Specific nutrients for detoxification:

- Vitamin B12
- Folic Acid
- Vitamin B6
- Methionine
- Vitamin A
- Magnesium
- Taurine
- Cysteine
- Glycine
- Selenium
- Potassium sulphate
- Inositol
- Choline bitartrate

Naturopaths have formulas that contain a combination of these herbs, vegetables, and nutrients. Often you can get them in one formula, or in some cases two separate formulas might be more beneficial for a certain individual.

An example of a good general liver formula might be something like this:

St Mary's thistle, schizandra, globe artichoke, broccoli, turmeric, taurine, glycine, vitamin B12, folic acid.

Once taken at therapeutic doses for at least two weeks, a liver formula may be taken at a maintenance dose over the long term if necessary, to enhance detoxification and improve hormonal balance. It is not recommended to take a liver formula without first doing stage one and two of a detox program. This is because if you have leaky gut syndrome, the toxins that the liver excretes through the bile will just be reabsorbed into the bloodstream. Healing the increased intestinal permeability first, allows the digestive tract to provide a good barrier to unwanted substances.

You may like to repeat this detox program again every six to twelve months to keep things on track and prevent toxic build up again. If you are prone to constipation, it might be a good idea to use the oxygen colon cleanser periodically, either once or twice a week, or do a six day course every two to three months.

After detoxing, many people often find that various niggling symptoms just disappear. Symptoms such as; headaches, bloating, bad breath, mood swings, stomach cramps and wind, acne, fatigue, and joint aches. It just goes to show how many things can result from toxic overload and a sluggish digestive system.

I have had patients come to see me for trouble conceiving, and once they performed a proper detox program involving the steps I've just outlined, they were able to become pregnant naturally. The body needs a strong, clean foundation for things to work efficiently. Proper detoxification and adequate nutritional intake helps to provide that strong foundation.

STEP FIVE: SUPPLEMENTATION

BASIC SUGGESTIONS FOR OPTIMAL HEALTH

- **Good quality multivitamin and mineral formula:**

Everyone should be taking a multivitamin. Because of the reduced supply of essential nutrients in the modern diet, we need to supplement if we want to improve our health. Remember, even if you eat a good diet, you may not be getting enough of everything you need. If it's not in the soil, it's not in the food.

There are too many multivitamins on the market, some expensive, some cheap. Usually, but not always, you get what you pay for. Cheaper formulas use cheaper synthetic ingredients that are not well absorbed or utilised by the body. Why pay for something that your body can't use?

There are two main types of quality multivitamins:

1. Standardised plant based or wholefood supplements that naturally contain vitamins and minerals.

2. Individual nutrients from natural sources combined in a formula in synergistic ratios.

Standardised means that what is written on the label is what you get. For example, you might have a supplement with a certain herbal ingredient, but you don't know whether the active ingredient is still present in that herb unless it is standardised. Plant based or wholefood supplements are usually a certain plant or combination of plants in their natural form that have been formed into a concentrated extract. Plant based formulas are always better absorbed and utilised than those produced synthetically, but standardisation is the key.

Other formulas that are combinations of nutrients can still be well utilised if they are formulated in ratios that optimise the absorption of each nutrient. Some nutrients, especially minerals, counteract each other when taken at the same time (e.g.: iron and calcium), and others help with the absorption of other nutrients (e.g.: vitamin C and iron), so a good quality formula will be made with this in mind. One way to check is to look at the amounts of each nutrient on the label. If all the minerals are rounded even numbers, then the formula may not have been made with much precision. Usually the amounts of some minerals should look like this – 67mg, 83.8mg, 40.4mg, 15.7mg, 102mcg…etc. Rather than 60mg, 80mg, 40mg, 15mg, 100mcg.

The rules about multivitamins are:

~ If getting a plant based formula, tablets or capsules are better than liquids or juices, and make sure it contains standardised vitamins and minerals, and preferably 'vitamin complexes' and phytochemicals. Usually with plant based formulas, one tablet a day is not enough as you can't fit everything you need into one tablet. Dosages might range from two to four tablets daily.

~ If getting a formulated nutrient combination, make sure the vitamin E it contains is natural. It should read; 'd-alpha-tocopherol', and not 'dl-alpha-tocopherol', as the synthetic form has been linked to health problems.

Make sure the amounts of B vitamins are high enough. Some good examples are: vitamin B1 – 50mg, vitamin B2 – 20mg, vitamin B3 – 100mg, vitamin B5 – 50mg, vitamin B6 – 40mg, vitamin B12 – 400mcg, folic acid – 400mcg, biotin – 50mcg.

I see many patients who have come to me taking cheaper formulas containing B vitamins in amounts such as 1mg, 2mg...etc and say things like "Multivitamins don't make any difference, I'm still tired". When I point out that their formula is to blame and place them on a new one, many can't believe the difference!

Minerals such as calcium and magnesium should be mostly in absorbable forms like amino acid chelates and citrates, rather than oxides. Most good formulas usually contain a combination of forms.

So if you haven't already, get yourself a good multivitamin formula!

- **Essential Fatty Acids:**

Many people don't get enough essential fatty acids, especially omega-3, in their diet, and because one of the highest sources is fish, there are concerns about eating too much because of the risk of mercury contamination.

These fats are essential, your body cannot make them, and they are vital for every cell in your body. They form cell membranes, and if you remember from section two, cell membranes are what allow stimuli from a cell's environment to make changes inside the cell. Any disruption to the membrane structure will affect a cell's function.

Omega-3 fats have anti-inflammatory properties. If you have PCOS you are almost definitely experiencing some degree of low grade chronic inflammation (even if blood tests say you aren't!). We are living in an inflammatory world – high intake of refined foods, high meat and dairy intakes, low fish and vegetable intake, stressful lifestyles, all these things contribute to your inflammatory load. Taking an omega-3 supplement is a good way of reducing this inflammatory load, as well as providing numerous other benefits for your hormones, metabolism, brain function, and memory. There may also be some risk reducing benefits in relation to cholesterol levels, blood pressure, and heart disease.

Fish oil is usually the best way to get extra essential omega 3 fats, but you need to take a good quality one to make sure you don't get more than you bargained for (like mercury!). Different countries have different standards that must be adhered to for a fish oil to be sold on the shelf. In some countries, including Australia, this standard is okay but not that high, as not all contaminants are tested for. I prefer to use companies that go beyond the standard, and voluntarily test their products for other contaminants such as pesticide residues and dioxins, and take steps to remove these contaminants.

Some people experience reflux or a fishy aftertaste on fish oils. My suggestion is to try some different brands, but make sure the brand is good quality and has an 'enteric coating' on it, which means it will not break down in the stomach, it will only digest once it reaches the intestines. Also, many over the counter fish oils have about half the active ingredients as some other brands, so don't just look for how much 'fish oil' is in the capsule (usually 1000mg), look at how much EPA and DHA is present. Most high quality fish oils should have around 300mg EPA, and 200mg DHA. That is what is important, not how much fish oil is present.

For vegetarians who don't eat fish, flaxseed oil can be used. It contains both omega-3 and omega-6 (and omega-9 which is not an essential fatty acid). However, fish oil usually provides more of an anti-inflammatory benefit as omega-6 fats have a 'pro-inflammatory effect'. They are still essential and beneficial, but it is when the balance is disrupted that problems begin. Most people get too much omega-6 and not enough omega-3. Spirulina can also be a good vegetarian source of essential fatty acids.

- **Glyconutrients:**

As you learned in section two, there are eight glyconutrients that the body uses each day for cellular communication. The different glyconutrients form different types of glycoproteins. The shape of the glycoproteins determines what kind of message is relayed to other cells and cell components. Glycoproteins also form molecules such as some hormones and enzymes, including the enzyme that allows your cells to reproduce.

We know they are vital for life, and that is why the body has a back-up system for manufacturing them, but we also know that this system uses up a lot of energy and nutrients, and is not always as efficient as needed due to toxins, stress, and nutrient deficiency. The body prefers to get these nutrients from a dietary source, but unfortunately due to modern farming practices, our food has become depleted in most of these nutrients (excluding glucose and galactose).

Due to the reduced availability in the food supply, and the limitations of biochemical conversion, I believe we should be supplementing with glyconutrients to optimise our overall health and improve cell communication processes in the body. Optimal communication equals optimal functioning, and optimal functioning equals optimal health!

The above three supplements nourish the cells, leading to better structure and function. They are the tools that provide a good base or framework for the body to work better.

ADVANCED SUGGESTIONS FOR OPTIMAL HEALTH

- **Antioxidants:**

To understand the significance of antioxidants, you must understand 'oxidative stress'. Every day during normal metabolism, your body produces molecules known as 'free radicals'. These molecules are unstable, they have an unpaired electron which causes them to 'take' electrons from other molecules, disrupting their structure. This is the process of oxidation.

In a state of optimal health, the body's oxidative processes don't cause ill health, but in some situations such as illness, inflammation, stress, intense exercise, nutritional deficiencies, and smoking, the oxidative processes in the body overwhelm the body's ability to deal with them and 'oxidative stress' results. This may cause damage to cells, and increase the likelihood of cellular dysfunction and premature ageing. This is where antioxidants come in.

Antioxidants, as their name implies, are 'against oxidation'. They help prevent free radicals from disrupting cells, by allowing free radicals to oxidise *them*. In a way, the antioxidant is sacrificing itself to protect other cells. They defend against oxidative stress, and help to maintain cellular structure and integrity. A cell that is protected will last longer and function effectively.

Choose an antioxidant supplement that has clinical research supporting its effectiveness, rather than just picking one up off the shelf. It is best to take a supplement that is natural, and contains a combination of plant ingredients rather than separate antioxidant nutrients added together in a formula. The plant's constituents work synergistically, and are usually more effective when used whole.

Many antioxidants are tested for effectiveness via the ORAC method (Oxygen Radical Absorption Capacity), which is an in vitro testing procedure. The supplement is then given an ORAC value, the higher the value, the more effective. This method only measures the antioxidant potential of *water soluble* molecules however, so the sORAC method, which tests the antioxidants in *serum* (a component of blood), is a more accurate predictor of how a supplement will work in the body. This is because it also tests fat soluble molecules, and your cells are made up of both fat and water soluble parts that both need protection.

Look for a supplement that has a high ORAC, or preferably, sORAC value, and make sure you check whether the value is per gram of supplement. For example, sometimes an antioxidant supplement will claim to have a high ORAC value, but the fine print says that it is per twenty grams. Divide the value by twenty and you may in fact have a low ORAC value!

- **Phytosterols:**

Phytosterols, including sitosterol, campesterol, and stigma-sterol, are also known as plant sterols, substances that can act as precursors to the body's steroid hormone production (eg: progesterone). Hormones are built from a series of precursors and intermediates, and some can also be converted to another (eg: testosterone can convert to oestrogen).

You might have heard about the benefits of phytosterols in relation to lowering cholesterol levels. They seem to reduce the absorption of cholesterol in the gut. There are many other benefits of phytosterols and research is still continuing in this area. An interesting study with rats showed that phytosterols actually resulted in a 33% decrease in testosterone levels. If this applies to humans it could be good news for women with PCOS[16].

Other effects may include a regulating effect on the immune system, anti-inflammatory effects, and helping with insulin production. By providing precursors for hormone production, they may benefit hormonal balance by allowing the body to produce hormones that are needed. They do not stimulate any specific hormone production, but simply provide the raw materials so the body can produce what it needs.

Phytosterols are mainly found in plant foods, especially pistachio nuts and sesame seeds. They are also in many vegetables and fruits, and wild yam is a particularly good source, but the same issues with modern farming practices and food processing apply, meaning that western countries may also be missing out on an optimal intake of phytosterols. It is interesting to observe that countries with high vegetable intakes and higher phytosterol intake tend to have less hormone related cancers, such as prostate and breast cancer, but more specific research needs to be done in this area.

Based on the positive benefits of phytosterols, and the reduction in supply in western countries, phytosterol supplementation may be a valuable addition to a supplement program for overall hormonal health.

- **Probiotics:**

As discussed in the detoxification section, probiotics are beneficial supplements that repopulate the gut with healthy bacteria. You will remember that many things in today's world upset the balance between good and bad bacteria, and can create an environment favourable to bacterial overgrowth. These things can include alcohol, processed foods, high GI foods, stress, antibiotic traces in the water supply, and certain medications.

We need beneficial gut flora to balance our immune systems, keeping inflammation at bay and reducing allergies and food intolerances. They can also protect against many gastrointestinal infections that cause vomiting and diarrhoea.

Beneficial bacteria are also particularly important when it comes to PCOS, because they act on soluble fibre in the digestive tract to produce short chain fatty acids like propionic acid, which stimulates sex hormone binding globulin (SHBG) production in the liver[17]. SHBG is needed to keep hormones like testosterone from acting upon cells, like your skin and hair.

Probiotics are essential during a detoxification program, but once the program is finished it can be a good idea to maintain a healthy gut flora with a maintenance probiotic formula. One that has both *lactobacillus* and *bifidobacterium* species is good, and make sure the amounts of bacteria are in the billions.

SPECIFIC SUPPLEMENTS FOR INDIVIDUAL SYMPTOMS

Although the aim of the 7 Step Solution is to deal with the underlying causes and bring about true healing, there are many symptomatic and specific treatments and therapies that can bring great results for various symptoms and associated conditions. These are discussed under the heading **'Targeted options for specific symptoms and conditions'**, just after step 7 in the 7 Step Solution.

These treatments can be implemented at the same time as the 7 steps if you like, to help target your symptoms more while you are making the necessary changes to your underlying state of health.

→See the resources page www.resources.poweroverpcos.com to find out where to get the natural supplements mentioned.

STEP SIX: MIND POWER

BASIC SUGGESTIONS

- **Schedule relaxation into your day:**

Stress can have a hugely negative impact on not only your PCOS symptoms, but your whole health, life, and relationships. Learning ways to respond rather than react to situations is important, to re-train your brain to be in a calm yet alert state.

When talking about stress management, it is not really stress that you are managing; it is *your perception* of stress.

Remember, your perceptions are one of the major factors that affect your health, by turning various genes on and off. Finding ways to change certain negative perceptions or replace them with positive perceptions will go a long way to improving your health.

Relaxation, however it is achieved, is one way of putting yourself in a state of mind that creates a positive perception. The point of relaxation is not to rest your body, but to balance your mind and connect with stillness. Stillness allows you to become more aware of your feelings and what is happening in your body, giving you greater insights and a feeling of control over your health and your life.

Achieving relaxation, where the body is still, the breathing is slow and deep, and the mind is calmly focused, can be brought about in a variety of ways. It doesn't matter which way you choose, just choose something that works for you. It is the relaxation response that is important, not how you achieve it. It usually works best when sustained for at least twenty minutes or more, but if you find ways of creating calm moments throughout your day you will still benefit.

You can achieve true relaxation by:

~ sitting still with your eyes closed, focusing on your breathing.
~ Lying down, focusing on one or two positive words or phrases.
~ Listening to a relaxation CD.
~ Taking a bath in candlelight, focusing on the feeling of lightness and a floating sensation.
~ Having a relaxation massage

After true relaxation you will feel refreshed, calm, and rejuvenated.

- **Deliberate affirmations:**

The words you use directly affect your state of mind, so choose them carefully. Words come from thoughts, conscious or unconscious, and thoughts are a form of energy. Remember that energy directly affects your cells and your genes, so your words can create changes in your body.

You can use this to your advantage by deliberately choosing positive words and statements. The best way to do this is to write some down, carry one or two with you each day, and repeat them several times daily, especially on waking and before sleep. These are called affirmations.

Affirmations should be said in the present tense, and they should describe and ideal feeling or situation in a way that is believable. For example, if you are trying to lose weight but every time you look in the mirror you feel unhappy and mutter negative words to yourself, try saying something positive but believable. You wouldn't say "I love my slim toned body" if you don't have a slim toned body. Your body will think "Yeah right!", and it will create a negative feeling which will be counterproductive. You need to feel good about your affirmation. Instead you could try "I love nurturing my body with a healthy diet and lifestyle".

Other affirmations you could try are:

~ I sleep soundly and wake feeling restored

~ I am loved and supported every day of my life

~ I have the power to create my life

~ I love feeling my body getting healthier every day

~ My body was designed to function in harmony

~ I choose to feel positive and happy in this moment

~ My skin has amazing healing ability

~ My life is a gift

- **Self Improvement through reading:**

Achieving a positive mindset is not like reaching the top of a mountain and then stopping. It is a continual journey of self improvement, and the more you take opportunities for self improvement, the more you will grow.

Reading books that educate, motivate, and inspire is one way of encouraging a greater understanding of how your mind works, and how you can improve your mindset and attitude to life and its challenges. There are many great books available that offer you new perspectives and ideas, and can help you lead a richer more fulfilling life. Make it a point to read a new inspiring book every few months, if not more frequently. Expand your mind and be open to opportunities for self improvement, and all areas of your life will benefit.

ADVANCED SUGGESTIONS

- **Meditation and Visualisation:**

Meditation is the art of relaxing your mind and body by focusing on one or two things. Often our minds are so cluttered with the busyness of daily life, it is easy to become accustomed to this as the default state of mind, but really, a calm focus should be the default state of mind, allowing us to see with clarity how things really are, and not be affected by past and future. It is about being in the present, because the present is all there is!

To really benefit, you can incorporate structured meditation into your life, preferably on a daily basis. Try twenty minutes each day, whether that be all in one go, or ten minutes on rising, and ten minutes before bed.

You can either have complete silence, use repetitive relaxation music, or use a guided meditation CD. Make it a ritual in your day, as important as having a shower and brushing your teeth, and you will start to see the benefits permeate your whole life.

For even greater benefits in regards to affecting your health, use visualisation. This is simply creating pictures in the mind's eye, of the way you would like things to be. You can spend a certain amount of time just visualising, or you can even do mini visualizations as you do your daily tasks.

Some examples of visualisations:

~ While having a shower, visualise the water washing away all toxins, and notice a new feeling of cleanliness inside. Imagine a healthy glow coming from inside, and all organs working perfectly.

~ During your cycle, visualise the egg forming perfectly in your ovary, and releasing effortlessly during ovulation. Repeat affirmations such as "My body is in a state of harmony and balance".

~ While exercising, visualise your muscles contracting and working efficiently, visualise sugar molecules entering your cells with ease, and producing life-giving energy. Visualise yourself the way you would like to be.

~ While washing your face, visualise clear smooth skin, and say an affirmation like "I love having clear and radiant skin".

You get the idea? See how many you can come up with, and you'll probably find they'll make you feel so good inside!

- **Daily worksheets:**

Positive attitudes and perceptions can improve your health, but the effects are amplified when these thoughts are written down on paper. It's like it brings the thoughts into reality and makes them real.

An advanced strategy you can use is to write down a selection of positive statements each day and read them out. The key is to do it regularly. Once every two months is not enough, it's better than not at all, but it needs to be done regularly enough that it becomes a kind of habit. Habits can be hard to get rid of, and in this case that's a good thing! Writing statements down daily also trains your mind to become more positive as a way of life.

The more you focus on the positive, the more positive you'll get in your life, it's as simple as that. What about those people who have won the lottery twice, or the people that always seem to have things go their way? Or have you ever had 'one of those days' where everything goes wrong? People seem to get more of what they get, simply because of what they are focusing on.

What I suggest is having a folder, notebook, or journal of some kind and creating positive statement worksheets. Sometime each day, preferably morning, spend anywhere from five to fifteen minutes writing down various positive statements. You can write the same ones each day, or add new ones as you think of them. When writing goals, it is best to focus on no more than three of them at any one time, and it is best to repeat the same goal statements daily, rather than changing them too often.

Divide your page into three sections and fill in the blanks:

1. Evidence
2. Gratitude
3. My Ideal life

1. Write down three or more good things that happened to you yesterday:

E.g.:
~ I had a great lunch out
~ I received a compliment
~ I had money left over after paying bills.
If you can't think of anything, get back to basics. E.g.: I was able to wake up and breathe.

2. Write down three or more things you are grateful for:

E.g.:
~ I am grateful for my family
~ I am grateful I have weekends off
~ I am grateful I saw the sunset last night.

3. Write three or more goals or affirmations that describe specific aspects of your ideal life: (be specific with time and dates, and focus on benefits)

E.g.:
~ I love knowing that my regular exercise routine I do on Mondays Wednesdays and Fridays is giving me a strong, toned, and slim body.
~ It is October 2009 (write a future date) and I'm extremely grateful that I'm now ready and able to become a mother.
~ I love looking in the mirror and feeling happy and confident within myself. My friends and family have noticed the positive change in me.

These daily worksheets really help in all aspects of your life. They are particularly useful when you are trying to achieve a specific goal. They work best when you really feel the benefits emotionally of what you are writing.

- **Release negative limiting beliefs:**

Most of us have belief systems that we have been brought up with, that are ingrained into our lives often unknowingly. Usually these beliefs stem from our childhood, when we were like a sponge, soaking up life, and taking on board the behaviours and habits that the people close to us followed.

Some of these may have been good, providing us with life skills that we use effectively today, and some may have been negative, causing us to be held back from certain things because of a belief that limits us. Eg: never being able to earn a good income because you were taught that "money doesn't grow on trees" and "rich people are selfish", or never having the courage to speak up for yourself because when you did you were criticised or judged.

Unknowingly, we shape our life and make choices based on our belief systems. But what if some of these belief systems are holding you back from achieving real health and happiness? What if those beliefs or perceptions are causing actual physical change in your body that is not congruent with health? Wouldn't you want to do what you can to change them so you can move forward?

There are certain techniques and professionals that can help you with releasing your internal saboteurs, those subconscious thoughts that stop you from achieving the results you want.

NLP, or neurolinguistic programming is one technique that can help. You can learn it through one on one sessions with an NLP practitioner, or you can do full NLP training yourself. NLP is based on how your mind and language connect to create your behavior. It can help you to reprogram your thoughts to ones that will serve you better. Details about NLP can be found at:
www.christopherhoward.info

Another technique that is having great results with releasing subconscious blockages is called PSYCH-K. It uses the practice of kinesiology or muscle testing to determine limiting beliefs and then works at changing those beliefs, often within minutes. It is quite amazing to watch it in progress. You can read about PSYCH-K at
www.psych-k.com

If you don't really know what your limiting beliefs are, let alone how to fix them, there are professionals that specialise in this area, by running workshops, online trainings, and one on one coaching.

Here are some I recommend:

www.beyondsuccess.com.au and
www.blockagebusters.com

There are also a few gifted people who are known as medical intuitives, those that can identify imbalances in the mind and body and often effect changes via an energy basis. If this is something you are interested in, contact POWER over PCOS.

STEP SEVEN: ACCOUNTABILITY AND SUPPORT

BASIC SUGGESTIONS

Social support:

Interaction with other people is an important part of a healthy lifestyle. Surround yourself with likeminded people and people who support you. Don't put up with negative and destructive relationships that don't serve you. Talk to others in a similar situation to yours, and remember, YOU ARE NOT ALONE. It can feel like it at times, but rest assured there are many others out there feeling the same desperation as you.

Have some form of positive social outlet, join a gym or sports club, a book club, go to seminars and talks, and chat with people in your neighbourhood. Call a friend, talk with supportive family members, and join an online support forum or local support group. Be there for others and let others be there for you. Focus on being around people that lift you up, people that inspire you and help to renew your hope. Although it can be good to get negative feelings off your chest, if you spend time with people who only talk about the negative, it will only exacerbate the problem. Remember, positivity helps to turn on those nourishing genes in your body.

Hold yourself accountable:

Accountability is having to 'check-in' with someone and report on what you have done or achieved for the past day, week, or month for example. Often, many people know what they need to do but don't do it for one reason or another. Having a system in place to provide accountability ensures that you will move closer and closer to your goals and achieve results.

To start with, you can hold yourself accountable. Schedule a time in your diary each day, week, or month (weekly is best) where you will sit quietly with yourself and ask yourself some questions. Treat this like an appointment with a coach, except in this case you are coaching yourself. If you have trouble sticking to something like this, then you may be better off enlisting the help of a coach who will encourage you to stick to your plan. You can also ask a good friend to help coach you, or maybe you could start an online 'accountability group' for women with PCOS to help each other stick to their goals.

If you are self disciplined however, then try coaching yourself and see how you go. Each week, ask yourself the following questions:

1. What did I do this past week to move myself closer to reaching my goals?

2. What obstacles were in my way this week?

3. How can I prevent these obstacles from getting in the way of reaching my goals?

4. How happy do I feel with my efforts this past week? (On a scale of 1 to 10)

5. What will I reward myself with at the end of the month if I stick to my plan?

6. What do I plan to do next week to move closer to better health and reaching my goals?

ADVANCED SUGGESTIONS

- **Get an accountability coach:**

The most successful people in business all have a coach or mentor. Why should it be any different when it comes to your health? Your health should be one of your top priorities, so you should pay it as much attention as you would a business. After all, to achieve a successful business you need to determine your goals, your resources, and create an action plan, as well as monitor and fine tune things as you go along. You can do the same with your health, and a coach can help you with this.

Even while writing this book I enlisted outside support to provide me with accountability, so I would get it finished in a reasonable amount of time. It had taken me three years to research, survey people with PCOS, try things on myself, and compile the general ideas and structure for this book. But when I committed to a system of accountability, I finished it all in six weeks, along with my online mentoring program at www.pcossuccess.com. I realised if I kept being a perfectionist it would never get finished, so I took action and stuck to a plan. It's amazing what you can achieve when you have someone on your back asking you "So, how much did you get done this week?"

Your coach can be someone who both gives you information on *what* to do as well as *how* to do it, or they can be someone who simply helps you do what you know you need to do.

Options for accountability:

1. Join up at www.pcossuccess.com and let me or a member of my team personally mentor you towards success. Whether you use this service for one month or twelve months, I can help you implement the advice in this book, and how to make it part of your life. The weekly email classes also act as an accountability tool as they guide you through the 7 step solution bit by bit.

2. See a qualified life coach to help you put the knowledge from this book into an action plan, and monitor your progress.

3. See a qualified naturopathic practitioner who is willing to work with you through the advice in this book, and provide ongoing support. *(As this book is being written, I am planning a certification course for health practitioners to train them in the Power Over PCOS protocol. I hope to build up a referral list of practitioners from different areas who will work through this program with you. To stay informed about this, make sure you subscribe to the PCOS newsletter at www.poweroverpcos.com).*

Remember, it's up to you!

If you want to achieve results, you have to take ACTION.

TARGETED OPTIONS FOR SPECIFIC SYMPTOMS AND CONDITIONS

- **Fat loss:**

In addition to the 7 Step Solution, there are some other things that can help to boost your fat loss:

~ Get the support of a coach:

People who have support during a fat loss program succeed more than those who don't. Buddy up with someone in the same position as you and help to motivate and inspire each other. Or, get a life coach or weight loss coach who can help keep you accountable. The email support as part of the membership program at www.pcossuccess.com is also designed to support and motivate you along your journey.

~ Substitute one meal or snack with a meal replacement:

When used properly, meal replacements can be very helpful as an adjunct to diet and exercise. They provide a balanced meal with the right ratios of protein, fats, and carbohydrates, and provide you with nutrients for your metabolism.

Meal replacements can be in the form of a drink or a bar. However, quality matters, so seek professional advice regarding the best formula for you.

~ Fibre mixture taken before meals:

If you are prone to feeling hungry a lot of the time, taking some fibre twenty minutes before a meal can help you to feel fuller, and less likely to overeat.

Soluble fibre when taken with water expands in the stomach as the fibre molecules take up water. This exerts some pressure on the walls of the digestive tract which stimulates the sensation of fullness in the brain. It also allows the muscles in your gut to work better, helping to prevent constipation.

Psyllium husks can help, but if you haven't used these before, start off with a small amount (1/2 tspn) to see how your body responds, and then increase gradually. Pectin and Slippery elm can also be beneficial. There are also some fibre mixtures that have been made for the purpose of creating the sense of fullness. Usually no more than one or two teaspoons is required for the effect, but it must be taken with a full glass of water.

~ Bitter melon:

Bitter melon can be beneficial for both weight loss and insulin resistance. It works by increasing the ability of cells to take up glucose, and this reduces the demand for insulin and allows more fat to be burned. It will also enhance the effects of exercise. Be aware that anything you take that can affect blood glucose control may increase the effects of some medications. Make sure you are monitored if combining any natural medicine with a drug like metformin.

~ Brown seaweed:

The brown seaweed *undaria pinnatifida* is showing promise in animal studies with regards to weight loss. A 10% decrease in weight was found in rats, and seems to be due to the ingredient fucoxanthin[18], which stimulates a protein in fat cells in the abdomen, causing an increase in metabolism and fat burning.

~ Green tea:

The catechins in green tea may have several health benefits, including stimulating metabolism and fat burning.

Remember, losing fat is about both biological factors and emotional/psychological factors. Long lasting success can only be achieved if you pay attention to both. Work on underlying limiting beliefs about your weight, and get support to deal with any emotional eating habits that may be present.

- **Insulin Resistance:**

The 7 Step Solution, especially the diet, lifestyle, and psychological factors will help with insulin resistance, but there are also some more specific things you can take to improve your insulin sensitivity.

~ Chromium:

Chromium is a trace mineral that allows insulin to attach to its receptor and bring glucose inside cells for energy. Insulin resistant people may need more chromium, and some studies have shown positive benefits with blood glucose control. A therapeutic dose would be a minimum of 200mcg daily (micrograms, not milligrams).

~ Magnesium:

Magnesium is also low in insulin resistant people, and I believe most people today are not getting enough as deficiency symptoms like leg cramps are very common. Magnesium helps insulin function and energy production, it also relaxes muscles and nerves. A therapeutic dose would be between 300mg and 800mg of 'elemental magnesium'.

~ Acacia and hops combination:

This is a very effective combination that can reduce both inflammation and insulin resistance, two major drivers of PCOS symptoms. Double blind animal studies show a 20% reduction in insulin levels, comparable to the effects of two mainstream anti-diabetic medications[19]. Human studies showed a 5% reduction in fasting insulin levels, and a 30% reduction in post-prandial insulin levels (2 hours after a glucose load)[20].

~ Gymnema sylvestre and Pterocarpus marsupium combination:

Like the acacia and hops formulation, this herbal combination has been shown in one study of 172 women with PCOS, to be as effective as metformin, without side effects[21].

~ alpha-lipoic acid:

Alpha-lipoic acid is well known for its benefits as an antioxidant. It also has beneficial effects on insulin resistance, including for people with diabetes. It seems to activate an enzyme called AMPK in muscle cells[22], which is responsible for activating glucose transporters that deliver glucose out of the bloodstream and into the cells. It is also known to significantly improve diabetic peripheral neuropathy at a dose of about 600mg daily[23].

~ apple cider vinegar:

Having some apple cider vinegar diluted in water before meals can be effective for lowering insulin levels.

- **Acne:**

If you are an acne sufferer, you may have been told that it's all due to an excess of male hormones. That's the truth but not the whole truth. You see, acne was always my main concern with PCOS, it was not unusual to have what seemed like fifty or so pimples, most of them cystic, which means they wouldn't come to a head and would last for weeks. They were painful, red, and ugly. There were times I wouldn't leave the house because of them, it affected my self esteem for years. The interesting thing was, my blood tests were all 'normal'. The male hormones were on the higher end of the range but not clinically abnormal, so if they were the cause of acne, why was my acne so bad and my hormones were classed as normal?

I discovered that acne was due to more than just hormones. A high glycaemic diet will increase acne, so I ate a low GI diet. Even when I was eating as healthily as possible, the acne was just as bad. I began to investigate the relationship between the health of the gut and the health of the skin.

The skin has many functions, one of which is as an elimination organ. If the gut and liver are overwhelmed, other organs compensate, including the skin. It wasn't until I did a detoxification program that my skin really started to improve. I also switched to natural skin care which has made a huge difference, and I became aware of negative thoughts about my skin and worked at changing them. Now, my skin is not perfect, but it is almost always 100% clear. I have scars, but it is great to look in the mirror and not see any active pimples. If I start to get a few minor ones, I know something in my lifestyle is out of whack, and I can usually pin point what it is, and then by correcting the imbalance my skin clears again.

So detoxification is vital, and so is a complete nutritional supplement program, especially essential fatty acids which regulate sebum (oil) production. Other factors to consider are:

~ Zinc:

Zinc is a common deficiency today, about 95% of people I test for zinc deficiency are deficient. In acne, zinc has been found to be helpful. It has many effects in the body, and may help acne by a combination of things such as balancing oil production, improving hormonal balance, helping skin healing, and improving immune function and the ability to fight bacteria in the skin.

The more zinc deficient you are, the less zinc you will be able to absorb from food and tablets, so a liquid zinc is usually the best form to replenish zinc levels as it is absorbed in a different way. Powders can also be useful.

It is best to get tested for zinc levels before supplementation. Taste tests (zinc tally) or hair analysis are useful. If you are an acne sufferer, depending on your level of deficiency, I would usually suggest a minimum of 30mg elemental zinc taken for about two months, or until a zinc tally shows improvement, then take either liquid or tablets every second day for another two months. You shouldn't take zinc in very high doses or for long periods of time, because it can interfere with the balance of other nutrients like copper.

~ Vitamin A:

Vitamin A is a fat soluble vitamin that regulates a variety of things in your body, including the rate of cell growth and healing. It helps the skin cells to mature and function properly, and allows them to slough off at the right time rather than building up and blocking the pores. The acne medication roaccutane actually has some resemblance to the function of vitamin A.

Vitamin A can build up in the body and cause damage to organs such as the liver, so high doses should not be taken without professional advice. Vitamin A can also be obtained by beta carotene, a natural pigment that gets converted to vitamin A in the body. Cod liver oil is a good source of vitamin A, and often it can be found in zinc supplements and multivitamins.

~ Vitamin B5:

Large doses of pantothenic acid have been used successfully with some acne sufferers. It seems to affect fat metabolism in the skin cells, reducing sebum excretion and pore size. Whenever any separate B vitamin is taken, it is always good to take a B complex or multivitamin as well.

~ Skin care:

Although acne is an outward symptom of an internal condition, what you put on your skin externally can also affect acne. If you use products that block the pores, acne is more likely to develop as there is nowhere for the oil to be eliminated and it backs up into the pores. Synthetic oil based products tend to be the worst offenders as they often sit on the external surface of the skin. Many natural oils are absorbed into the skin, so they are less likely to block the pores unless a lot is applied.

Natural skin care is best, it not only provides cleansing and hydration, but provides nutrients to the skin cells. Exfoliation is also important, to slough off dead skin cells and prevent pores getting blocked.

Natural skin care details can be found at:
www.resources.poweroverpcos.com

~ **Herbs:**

Herbal medicine can also be helpful for acne. I took herbs for years and they reduced my acne by about half. Good herbs include peony, licorice, chaste tree (vitex), burdock, St. Mary's thistle, Echinacea, golden seal, calendula. Also, use tea tree oil topically for breakouts, it will kill the bacteria and reduce the oil build up. Comfrey ointment and aloe vera can be used once the pimple has passed, to help healing and prevent scarring.

Chinese herbal medicine can also be especially effective for clearing acne, but remember, detoxification, nutrition, and the right mindset are vital.

- **Hair loss & Excess hair:**

These are both due to conversion of testosterone to more active androgens in the skin and hair follicles. Following the 7 Step Solution will naturally reduce your testosterone and provide you with nutrients necessary for healthy hair.

In addition, hair loss can be due to insufficient nutrients such as iron, folic acid, biotin, and essential fatty acids. Poor blood flow to the skin can also contribute. If you also get cold hands and feet easily, as well as hair loss, this could be a factor for you. Yoga poses that encourage blood flow to the skin and head area can be helpful, as can certain essential oils massaged into the scalp.

In addition to a basic nutritional program, extra biotin may be beneficial (about 300mcg), get your iron levels tested, make sure your multivitamin has a good amount of folic acid (a minimum of 400mcg), or supplement with a separate folic acid. Also, take fish or flaxseed oil for the essential fatty acids. Peony and licorice can help, as can the herb saw palmetto.

Also, try switching to a different shampoo and conditioner, one without sodium laureth sulfate. Some people find this exacerbates hair loss.

The use of essential oils (aromatherapy) has shown great results for reducing the amount of hair loss, and aiding in regrowth, but it takes a long time. One recipe that was used in studies is as follows:

1. Thyme essential oil - 2 drops
2. Atlas cedarwood essential oil - 2 drops
3. Lavender essential oil -3 drops
4. Rosemary essential oil -3 drops
5. Jojoba oil - ½ teaspoon
6. Grapeseed oil - 4 teaspoons

The mixture is massaged into the scalp each night for two minutes, and the head is wrapped in a towel.

More details can be found at:
www.stophairlossnow.co.uk/Aromatherapy.htm

- **Fertility:**

In addition to the 7 Step Solution, certain things can improve your chances of conception:

~ Acupuncture:

This complementary therapy has shown good results with improving ovulation rates in women with PCOS.

~ Visualisation and stress reduction:

Visualising yourself pregnant, or visualising yourself with a baby is a very good idea, as it keeps you focused on the outcome you wish to achieve, and not the problem of conceiving itself. Reducing your stress response can also help as it benefits your hormone balance, and creates a more favourable environment for conception.

~ Insulin sensitising agents:

As discussed under insulin resistance, these herbs can help fertility in PCOS by reducing the hormonal imbalance that comes from hyperinsulinaemia.

~ Weight loss treatments:

The methods discussed under weight loss will also help if you are overweight with PCOS. Losing just 5% of your weight can make a big difference. Fertility is hampered by being overweight, so every effort should be made to lose excess body fat, especially before considering fertility drugs.

~ Herbs:

Some beneficial herbs for increasing the likelihood of conception are; peony and licorice, chaste tree (especially if you have low progesterone and/or high prolactin), false unicorn root, dong quai, and wild yam. Chaste tree (*vitex agnus castus*) seems to work best when taken on rising, at least 500mg-1000mg daily. It also works best when other herbs are used as well, to give a more balanced effect on the hormones.

- ## Endometriosis & period pain:

~ Fish oil:

It reduces the anti-inflammatory prostaglandins which reduces pain. It also has regulatory effects on hormones.

~ Magnesium:

For its anti-spasmodic effects and anti-inflammatory effects.

~ Herbs:

Hops and turmeric combined have a good anti-inflammatory and pain relieving effect, and also an immune regulating effect. We know that endometriosis is associated with an immune imbalance. Hops also has the added benefit of reducing insulin resistance. Wild yam has anti-spasmodic effects and can be helpful for pain, and rosemary helps to reduce oestrogen dominance which is a part of endometriosis.

- **PMS/PMT – premenstrual syndrome:**

~ Magnesium:

Relaxes the nervous system, reducing anxiety. Helps with pain and inflammation.

~ Vitamin B6:

Has diuretic properties which have been shown to improve symptoms such as breast tenderness.

~ St. John's Wort:

Well known as an anti-depressant, when taken regularly it can help with chronic premenstrual tension involving episodes of anxiety and depression.

~ Zizyphus:

Has sedative and anti-anxiety effects. Can also help with premenstrual insomnia and heart palpitations.

~ Chaste tree:

Works well for many PMT symptoms, especially breast tenderness, acne, and mood swings.

Other useful herbs include wild yam, dong quai, passionflower, and withania.

- **Sugar and carbohydrate cravings:**

The treatments for insulin resistance will help here, especially gymnema sylvestre and chromium. Eating low GI is vital, and eating every two to three hours can help.

- **Underactive thyroid:**

This is usually due to either an autoimmune response (Hashimoto's thyroiditis), or a deficiency of nutrients like iodine. If the cause is not autoimmune, then nutritional supplementation should be tried first, before replacing the hormone artificially, unless it is a severe case. Other nutrients like tyrosine, selenium, and zinc are needed for thyroid hormone production. Kelp is a good source of iodine, but is best taken under professional supervision as in some cases it can worsen certain cases of hypothyroidism. It is best when diagnosed with hypothyroidism, to ask for a urinary iodine test, to see whether you are deficient. The herb *coleus forskolii* has also been used for many years as a thyroid stimulant.

- **High blood pressure:**

~ **Magnesium:**

Another condition where magnesium is beneficial! Magnesium helps relax the smooth muscle in the blood vessels, helping them to dilate and reducing the pressure of the blood against the vessel walls. Dosage should be a minimum of 400mg daily. Magnesium also helps the heart muscle to function better.

~ **Taurine:**

Works well with magnesium, especially for stress related high blood pressure. It acts on reducing sympathetic nervous stimulation, which has a relaxing effect.

~ Hawthorn:

A herb with tonic effects on the heart, and a vasodilatory action, which can lower blood pressure by creating more space in the blood vessels.

~ Bonito Peptides:

These are a type of protein found in the bonito fish, often consumed in Japan. Studies show they have natural blood pressure lowering effects, similar to ACE inhibitor drugs, which work by reducing constriction of blood vessels. They can also be taken alongside pharmaceutical blood pressure medication.

- **High cholesterol:**

~ Phytosterols:

As discussed as part of step 5, phytosterols help to lower cholesterol by reducing its absorption in the digestive tract.

~ Policosanols:

These are also known as sugar cane wax alcohols, and have been well researched, showing assistance with maintaining normal cholesterol levels. A dose of 10mg is needed.

~ Chinese red yeast rice:

Also known as *Oryza sativa,* red yeast rice has shown benefits in several studies. Overall it results in a reduction in cholesterol levels, but an increase in HDL levels (good cholesterol). It seems to work fairly quickly too (benefits documented at four weeks).

- **Headaches or migraines:**

Migraines are often associated with insulin resistance, inflammation, and food intolerances. Again, magnesium supplementation can help, along with coenzyme Q10, and the herb feverfew. Detecting any food intolerances is a good idea. They are often associated with intolerances to msg, salicylates, preservatives, wheat, and chemicals in wine and some cheeses.

For non-migraine headaches, dehydration is often a culprit, as is spinal misalignment, stress, and toxic overload.

- **Depression:**

~ **St John's Wort:**

A very effective anti-depressant, it works by increasing your nerve cell exposure to serotonin.

~ **Fish Oils:**

Omega 3 fats have shown benefits in regulating mood and behavior.

~ **SAMe (S-Adenosyl Methionine):**

This molecule is involved in the synthesis of various neurotransmitters in the brain, including serotonin. It should not be used by those with bipolar disorder as it may exacerbate a manic state in some people.

- **Anxiety:**

~ **Magnesium:**

Magnesium calms and slows down nervous system activity, which can help in cases of nervousness or anxiety.

~ **Herbs:**

There are many beneficial herbs for anxiety, including zizyphus, magnolia, and passionflower. Also, baical skullcap and valerian can be useful.

- **Irritable bowel syndrome:**

A detox program as outlined in the 7 Step Solution will almost certainly help, as will stress reduction and specific supplements like magnesium (surprise surprise!), slippery elm, and probiotics – *especially lactobacillus plantarum*. Avoiding wheat or gluten also helps a lot of people, and peppermint tea can be useful.

DEALING WITH SIDE EFFECTS IF YOU ARE ON MEDICATION

Following the 7 Step Solution and looking after your nutritional requirements will often reduce any side effects from medication, if you need to take them that is. Many of you reading this may already be taking medication, and so I have included some simple steps you can take to reduce certain side effects, and/or reduce the risks of the medication.

Metformin:

You must be on a good multivitamin, and a separate vitamin B12 and folic acid is recommended to maximise your intake, especially if you are trying to conceive. Monitor your B12 levels, and arrange for a B12 injection if necessary.

Probiotics may help reduce the stomach upset, as well as ginger. Ginger is used for nausea and is very effective. Try 500mg three times a day with meals. Slippery elm powder will also help with bowel upset. Take one or two teaspoons daily with plenty of water.

Birth Control Pills:

You must be on a good multivitamin, possibly some extra vitamin B6, folic acid, and magnesium. Chromium may help improve glucose tolerance, and the herb gymnema can reduce blood sugar swings. Zinc levels can become low, so get them checked or take a zinc supplement every second day.

Take essential fatty acids like fish oil, and eat lots of garlic, to reduce inflammation in the blood, and reduce the stickiness of the blood cells, as the pill can make you more prone to clotting.

The pill also reduces levels of good bacteria in the gut, so a probiotic supplement is vital. Take it at night before bed.

If you have been on the pill for a while, you may like to look at other options, as it is not the best treatment for PCOS over the long term because it makes insulin resistance worse.

Roaccutane:

Used for acne, this is a powerful drug that can have many side effects and risks. The first thing to be aware of is *not* to take supplemental vitamin A, as it can enhance the effects of the drug and lead to toxicity problems. You will need to find a multivitamin that only has beta-carotene as its vitamin A source, as this is a precursor for vitamin A that is water soluble and can be eliminated more easily. A plant based multivitamin formula would probably be your best bet.

Drink plenty of water and take essential fatty acids like fish or flaxseed oil to keep the skin moisturised from within. Roaccutane will give you very dry and flaky skin.

Use good quality natural skin care products. Your skin will absorb more moisture because of the dryness, and will be more likely to absorb certain chemicals from synthetic skin care, so natural is best. Apply moisturiser regularly throughout the day to prevent excessive dryness. Use a body cream after each shower, and carry a hand cream with you at all times to use after washing your hands, or they will become red and sore.

Use slippery elm powder daily to soothe dryness in the intestinal tract and to prevent pain and anal tears when moving your bowels.

Consider a herbal liver formula to help reduce the risk of liver complications. St Mary's thistle is a good herb to use.

Antibiotics:

Antibiotics, often used for acne, will kill off good bacteria in your digestive tract and other areas of the body, and make you more prone to digestive upsets and thrush. While on antibiotics, take the beneficial yeast *sacchoromyces boulardii* (SB) which can reduce the incidence of antibiotic associated diarrhea and thrush. Take a break from SB for about a week, after every twelve weeks of supplementation to allow it to shed.

You can take probiotics as well, but the antibiotics will kill them off so it can be a waste of money, but if you take them at least four hours away from the antibiotics, you can obtain some benefit that may be enough to prevent side effects for a certain amount of time. For example, if taking antibiotics twice a day, take them at breakfast and lunch, and take the probiotics before bed. When you finish your antibiotic course, take a course of high dose multi species probiotics for at least a couple of months.

IMPLEMENTING THE 7 STEP SOLUTION

Once you have read the 7 Step Solution, it is a good idea to make a plan of how you will implement it. Go through each step and highlight or write down the things that you are ready to take on board.

To give you an idea, I have included a written plan of the main things I have done to achieve success:

My program:

My program changes here and there, and some things I do periodically, but to give you an idea of how I achieved success, this is what I found worked for me:

Step 1: Diet & Nutrition

- Low GI diet.

- Healthy, balanced, natural foods diet. Red meat no more than twice per week.

- Organic vegetables and meats whenever possible.

- Plenty of water, no coffee or tea except dandelion, when having juice I dilute it half with water.

- No dairy or gluten. Occasionally I'll have some, but if I eat these foods regularly my symptoms start to resurface.

- I identified my food allergies and intolerances. Avoid foods with allergic reactions, avoid some foods with inflammatory reactions, reduce the intake of others to only occasionally.

- Occasionally when eating out or on special occasions, I will have small amounts of dairy and wheat. I never eat these foods however without first taking a special enzyme supplement. One that breaks down the bonds between the amino acids of these foods, to reduce the amount of beta-casomorphin and gliadamorphin absorbed. I also take the probiotic lactobacillus plantarum for a few days afterwards to reduce any inflammation that may be produced in the gut.

- My usual daily menu:

Breakfast:	- gluten free muesli (rice bran, rice puffs, buckwheat, almonds, dried strawberry, chickpeas, raisins, sunflower seeds), with protein enriched rice milk. I also sprinkle on 1 dessertspoon of LSA mix, and a fibre mixture (pectin, aloe vera, slippery elm, glutamine). - Diluted juice. - Nutrient supplements
Snack:	- Fruit such as mandarin, nectarine, grapes, or a dried

	fruit bar. - cashew nuts
Lunch:	- Omelette with mushrooms, Spanish onion, and spinach leaves. OR - Salad with spinach leaves, carrot, capsicum, avocado, walnuts, and either chicken or salmon. Olive oil dressing. OR - Low GI gluten free sandwich with salmon and avocado and salad, or natural peanut butter when in a hurry. -Nutrient supplements
Snack:	- homemade low GI gluten free muffin, or seed crackers and hummous
Dinner:	- meat, chicken, or fish with stir fried mushrooms and bok choy with mustard dressing. OR - Vegetable soup OR Meat, chicken, or fish with mashed sweet potato and vegetables - Nutrient supplements

Step 2: Exercise

- I used to do two dance classes a week, as well as planning classes and choreography for several hours each week.

- When wanting to lose weight I did extra exercise like walking, for 20-30 minutes four times a week, plus resistance training for 30 minutes every 2nd or 3rd day.

- Now I do lots of incidental exercise, I walk quickly when I shop, I move around while on the phone, and I stretch several times throughout the day. My exercise schedule varies, but generally it is based around resistance exercise – working on one major muscle group each day for about 10 minutes (upper body, abdominals, lower body), walking on the treadmill or out and about, and yoga stretches before bed.

Step 3: Lifestyle & Complementary Therapies

No smoking, no alcohol, one hour for lunch each day, making time for relaxation. Occasional massages and osteopathic adjustments. I also spent a year doing acupuncture every few weeks, which helped with hormonal balance and stress.

Step 4: Detoxification

I use natural products wherever possible, and I do a detoxification program every 3 to 6 months.

Step 5: Supplementation

This has changed over the years, and some things I take courses of periodically, but this is generally what I take at the time of writing this book:

- Plant based multivitamin, 3 - 4 tablets daily.

- Antioxidant formula with a sORAC score of over 17,000. 2 capsules daily.

- Wild yam and phytosterol supplement. 3 tablets daily.

- Glyconutrients powder. 2-4 tspns daily.

- Probiotic formula, 1 capsule daily

- Magnesium, 300-400mg daily.

- Vitamin B12 and folic acid, 1 tablet every second day.

- Ultra Clean Fish Oil, 3 capsules daily.

- Acacia and Hops herbal formula. 2-3 capsules daily.

This may seem like a lot to some of you, but I wouldn't be without them. I have seen my health improve greatly through supplementation, and I am interested in being proactive, acting on the available research into nutritional deficiencies of modern lifestyle, and investing in preventative health care. Health is one of your most important assets, without it, you can't enjoy your life fully.

Step 6: Mind Power

Most days, I spend about fifteen minutes writing down positive statements. Things I am grateful for, good things that have happened, and my goals and desires.

I visualise often, I listen to meditation CD's, and I watch inspirational DVD's. I rarely watch the news as it just adds to negativity, once a week is enough to stay informed.

I use affirmations, and place affirmation cards under my pillow at night. I read inspirational and self improvement books, and I attend self improvement workshops and seminars, to continue to allow myself to grow.

I never go to bed with a negative emotion if I can help it. I try and reframe my state of mind to a positive one before sleep, and focus on the intention I have for the next day. Most of all, I just try to be thankful for the life I have, keep reminding myself of all the good things in life, and aim to experience joy every day.

IN CONCLUSION:

From my heart to yours, I would like to wish you the very best in your journey. Remember that you have an amazing healing ability inside of you that is waiting for you to activate it. This book has given you the knowledge and tools to transform your health, and now it is up to you to take action, to turn the knowledge into results. Are you ready? Go for it!

For further support with PCOS, please see the 'Resources' page overleaf.

RESOURCES

- The PCOS Success System online program: www.pcossuccess.com*

  *As a special bonus for buying this book, you are entitled to a trial of my online membership program for only $1 for thirty days.
  Please visit the following webpage for details:
  www.poweroverpcos.com/bonusmembership.html

- Keep up to date with my PCOS tips and news, as well as receiving the free A-Z of PCOS email course, at www.poweroverpcos.com

- For recommended products as mentioned in this book, visit the resources webpage at:
  www.resources.poweroverpcos.com

- Are you a health professional? For details of becoming a certified Power Over PCOS Practitioner, please visit:
  www.poweroverpcos.com/practitioners.html

- For wholesale/bulk orders of this book, please visit:
  www.poweroverpcos.com/wholesale.html

- PCOS Support Associations:
  Australia: www.posaa.asn.au
  USA: www.pcosupport.org
  UK: www.verity-pcos.org.uk

- Please direct all enquiries regarding this book or the author to: info@poweroverpcos.com

REFERENCES

1. Regan, L, et al. Hypersecretion of LH, infertility and spontaneous abortion. Lancet 336 (8724), 1990: 1141-44

2. http://www.abc.net.au/news/stories/2008/01/22/2144176.htm . Quoting research published in the American Journal of Obstetrics and Gynaecology.

3. MIMS Australia 1993. MediMedia Australia Pty Ltd NSW.
3. Osiecki, H. The Physicians Handbook Of Clinical Nutrition. 5th edn. 1998. Bioconcepts Publishing. QLD. Australia.
3. Braun, L, & Cohen, M. Herbs & Natural Supplements, An Evidence Based Guide. 2005. Elsevier Mosby. NSW. Australia.

4. Anderson, R.N. National Vital Statistics Report. Volume 50, Number 16. Sept 16, 2002.
http://www.cdc.gov/nchs/data/nvsr/nvsr50/nvsr50_16.pdf

5. Starfield, B. JAMA – Journal of The American Medical Association. July 26, 2000;284(4):483-5
http://www.ncbi.nlm.nih.gov/pubmed/10904513?dopt=Abstract

6. Nugent, S. How To Survive On A Toxic Planet. 2nd edn. 2006. The Alethia Corporation. USA.

7. http://www.non-toxic.info/Health_Statistics.htm

8. Handa, O, et al. 'Methylparaben potentiates UV-induced damage of skin keratinocytes'. Toxicology. 2006 Oct 3;227(1-2):62–72. Epub 2006 Jul 28.
http://www.ncbi.nlm.nih.gov/sites/entrez

9. Darbre, P.D, et al. 'Concentrations of parabens in human breast tumours', Journal Of Applied Toxicology. Volume 24 issue 1 pp 5-13.
http://www3.interscience.wiley.com/journal/106600317/abstract

10. Nugent, S. How To Survive On A Toxic Planet. 2nd edn. 2006. The Alethia Corporation. USA.

11. Fenkci, V, et al. 'Decreased total antioxidant status and increased oxidative stress in women with polycystic ovary syndrome may contribute to the risk of cardiovascular diseas'e. Fertility and Sterility. 2003 Jul;80(1):123-7.
http://www.ncbi.nlm.nih.gov/pubmed/12849813

12. Rich-Edwards, JW, et al. Milk consumption and the pre-pubertal somatotropic axis. Nutrition Journal. 2007 Sep 27;6:28.
http://www.ncbi.nlm.nih.gov/pubmed/17900364

13. Berker, B. 'Increased insulin like growth factor-1 levels in women with polycystic ovary syndrome, and beneficial effects of metformin therapy'. Gynecology & Endocrinology. 2004, Sep;19(3):125-33.

14. Woodford, Keith. Devil In The Milk. 2007. Craig Potton Publishing, New Zealand).

15. Lack of sleep hurts women's hearts most:
http://www.medicinenet.com/script/main/art.asp?articlekey=88021

16. Taheri, S, et al. 'Short Sleep Duration Is Associated with Reduced Leptin, Elevated Ghrelin, and Increased Body Mass Index'.
http://www.pubmedcentral.nih.gov/articlerender.fcgi?artid=535701

17. http://www.buffalo.edu/news/3460

18. Hungerford, C. Good Health In The 21st Century – a family doctor's unconventional guide. 2006. Scribe Publications Pty Ltd, VIC, Australia.

19. http://nutraingredients-usa.com/news/ng.asp?id=70505

20. Lerman RH, Tripp ML, Bland JS. Effects of Hops/Acacia supplementation in overweight subjects with insulin resistance. Draft report submitted for publication. Received January 2007.

21. Lerman RH, Tripp ML, Bland JS. Effects of Hops/Acacia supplementation in overweight subjects with insulin resistance. Draft report submitted for publication. Received January 2007.

22. http://humrep.oxfordjournals.org/cgi/reprint/21/suppl_1/i177.pdf

23. Je Lee, et al. Biochemical and Biophysical Research Communications, Volume 332, Issue 3, 8 July 2005 pp 885 – 891. Link: doi:10.1016/j.bbrc.2005.05.035

24. http://www.ncbi.nlm.nih.gov/pubmed/17065669

CPSIA information can be obtained at www.ICGtesting.com
Printed in the USA
LVOW071326280213

322118LV00007B/46/P

9 781921 681356